Ministering
to the Hurting

Women's Mental Health and
Pastoral Response in Ghana

Angela Dwamena-Aboagye

First published by March in 2021

ISBN: 978 – 9988 – 3 – 1933 – 5

PRODUCED IN GHANA

Typeset & Printed by University of Ghana Printing Press, Legon P. O. Box LG 1181 Legon, Accra, Ghana Email: ugpress@ug.edu.gh

DEDICATION

To the Triune God alone, Father, Son and Holy Spirit (Agya Pa, me Gyefo
ne me Nua Panin Yesu, m'Adanfo Pa ne Boafoɔ Homhom Kronkron), I
never could have made it without You.

The Lord has promised good to me
His Word my hope secures
He will my shield and portion be
As long as life endures...*

*(John Newton, 1725-1807: Ancient and Modern,
Third verse of the hymn 'Amazing Grace')

ACKNOWLEDGMENTS

I am deeply grateful to Almighty God who accompanied me on the journey of studying for my doctorate. He was my Strength, Wisdom, Provider, Comfort and Healer, time and again. He provided me with remarkable people who supported me with resources I cannot quantify.

One of such is my greatest cheerleader, my mother, Rose Dua-Sakyi, who passed away on August 1, 2017, at the age of 94. She would have read my whole thesis had she been here when I completed!

I am very grateful for Professor Allison Howell, my primary doctoral supervisor under whose tutelage my writing and research skills vastly improved. Her constant encouragement to have me publish is what has led to the actualization of this project. I am also grateful to Dr Araba Sefa-Dedeh and Rev Dr Ernestina Afriyie, my additional supervisors, for their helpful comments and encouragement.

I also wish to thank Professor Emeritus Andrew F. Walls who granted me a very interesting interview during the research period. It is a joy to know that a man who is easily described as a 'walking encyclopaedia' of Church History and Mission Studies, Andrew Walls, is not only my teacher, but contributed to my thesis!

I also wish to show my appreciation to all others who participated in, and in any way contributed to the shaping of this work. I wish to mention in particular:

ACI staff, especially Mr Ben Asiedu (Uncle Ben), McWilliams Hodzi and the other Zimmermann Library staff, and Yaw Agyemang (Wofa Yaw) whose warm welcoming smiles, help and encouragement cheered me up whenever I went to the ACI campus;

MindFreedom and BasicNeeds Ghana, led by Mr Dan Taylor and Mr Peter Yaro respectively;

Dr Akwasi Owusu Osei, Executive Secretary of Mental Health Authority and Dr Ama Edwin, Medical Doctor, Bio-Ethicist and Clinical Psychologist;

Dr Evangelist Ebenezer Abboah-Offei of the Presbyterian Church of Ghana (PCG), Akropong and Patmos Christian Centre; Mrs Theresa Wiafe-Asante, Family Life Counsellor, International Central Gospel Church (ICGC), Liberty Temple, Ashongman, Accra;

Dr Cephas Narh, Director, Vision and Legacy, Head Office, ICGC Miotso; Rev Dickson Sarpong Tuffour, ICGC Jesus Temple, Koforidua, and Rev Samuel Wiafe Asante, ICGC Liberty Temple, whose encouraging words and sermons made me believe, indeed, that 'He who has begun a good work in me is also able to bring me to its completion...';

The Rectors of Pentecost Theological Seminary (PTS) and Daniel Institute of ICGC, the President of Trinity Theological Seminary (TTS), Senior officials of the headquarters of Church of Pentecost (COP), Ghana; Assemblies of God (AOG), Ghana; Presbyterian Church of Ghana (PCG) and International Central Gospel Church (ICGC), without whom I could not have done this work:

Also, heads and officials of the Pantang Hospital, Accra Psychiatric Hospital and the Department of Psychiatry of the University of Ghana Medical School (UGMS), Korle-Bu;

The 20 Pastors I interviewed from the four denominations;

The 10 Christian women survivors I interviewed: my sisters-in-Christ and 'in arms';

Rev Professor Abraham Adu Berinyuu of Tamale, who encouraged me a great deal;

Mrs Griselda Lartey of Columbia Theological Seminary Library, Atlanta, Georgia, USA;

Edwin Boakye-Yiadom, Clinical Psychologist and Dunstan Akoto, Research Assistant, who helped me with transcribing and coding data; Dr Akosua Darkwa, Department of Sociology, University of Ghana, who helped me gain a better understanding of qualitative research;

Dr Maureen O. Iheanacho, an excellent editor of this work and a great encourager;

My own church family the congregation of ICGC Liberty Temple, Atomic Hills, Ashongman, Accra. Your prayers work!

My sister-friend–Jane Quaye; my dear niece Dr. Aba-Sah Dadzie who gave me a hiding place to write in faraway Scotland, and the many others near and abroad who simply cheered me on...

My natal family, the Dua-Sakyis and our many descendants, who bring to me the enduring qualities of much laughter and many debates that have greatly shaped who I am today. Those breaks with my family during my writing were so refreshing, providing the much needed 'boost' to return to my laptop and keep going!

Finally, to my dear husband, Kwame, who kept encouraging me to 'hurry up, finish and publish'. You are like a pillar and I thank God for you! To my dear children, Freda, Dorsina, Nana Akua and Papa K., and to Aiden Angelo and Ryan, my grandchildren, thank you for being there. God bless you all!

FOREWORD

It is my privilege to share a few reflections on this insightful study by Dr. Angela Dwamena-Aboagye. This important publication comes from a section of her PhD thesis on Women's Mental Health and the Pastoral Response. It is not only a welcome event but also reflects groundbreaking research in the way Dr. Dwamena-Aboagye deftly discusses these two facets of the Ghanaian Christian experience. Although in the West there are many studies on different aspects of mental health and illness, far fewer have been carried out in Africa. In spite of all the available literature and the plethora of materials especially online on mental health and well-being and the increase of material during the Covid-19 pandemic, scholarly and practical evidence of how pastors respond to women's mental health has been neglected. The twin problems of associated stigma and lack of understanding of mental health issues permeate all societies in the world. They are also particularly apparent in African societies.

The late twentieth and early twenty-first centuries have evidenced a rapid growth of churches in many African countries, including Ghana. In most of these churches, women predominate. Pastors of these churches are expected to interact with their members significantly women who face various difficulties, including unrecognised, undiagnosed and misunderstood mental distress and illness. As Dr. Dwamena-Aboagye points out, Christian women tend to first seek out their pastors for counsel and prayer when problems arise because the women perceive the pastors to be the link between their faith and God's intervention in their situations.

In the fascinating study which follows, Dr. Dwamena-Aboagye elucidates the critical role of pastors in responding to those who are suffering in the church. Yet, dire problems persist because of a serious lack of knowledge and understanding of mental health on the part of pastors and religious leaders. At the outset of the study, Dr. Dwamena-Aboagye states her motivation for embarking on the research that led to this book. It is in that context that she provides her own experience.

During the research for this work, Angela experienced, at times, deep mental and emotional stress. As one of her supervisors, I struggled with not knowing how to balance the mental pressure I was placing on her to complete her fieldwork across Ghana and the research in general. I found myself constantly asking, "Is this too much for her to bear?" I recall a lengthy telephone call she made from a remote part of Ghana to me in Akropong-Akuapem during which we discussed the need to adjust the exigencies of the research and for her to have a break to recoup her strength before continuing with the research. That she completed this research is testimony to her resilient faith in God and to the lessons she garnered from her experiences which helped her manage the stress.

Dr. Dwamena-Aboagye is therefore well equipped as an interpreter of the mental health indicators she discovered in her research. As she points out, she is herself a survivor of mental illness. This means that she writes not only as a researcher and participant-observer, but more importantly also as an insider who experienced the mishandling of her own mental health challenges by some well-meaning pastors.

While providing background material, chapters three, four and five cover a general overview of women, gender and mental health; Christian women coping with mental health and the role of the church; and mental health in Ghana. Some definitions of important terms helpfully guide the reader throughout the work.

The core of Dr. Dwamena-Aboagye's research is however located in chapters six to eight. There she juxtaposes the experiences of Ghanaian Christian women facing mental health challenges as well as their perspectives on responses, with the actual pastoral responses they received. The women's responses are illuminating as they help to break stereotypes about how women respond to mental and emotional challenges. The pastors' responses invite a closer examination and point to the need for further research in this area. Under the apt title, 'A Call to do Justice and Show Mercy', Dr. Dwamena-Aboagye draws together the findings and far-reaching implications of the study.

This book has been written for the benefit of us all. It is for all women and men who want to understand their personal mental health issues and need encouragement in how to relate to them. I highly recommend it particularly to all pastors and to those in positions of social responsibility who desire, like Christ, to minister to the hurting and who are humble enough to acknowledge that not all mental and emotional issues have solely spiritual causes.

More studies like this one are needed to help deepen our understanding of the mental health issues that many people face and the crucial role that pastors, Christians, the Church and mental health professionals can and should play in alleviating the suffering of many women and men in our societies. In the meantime, we can welcome and read this work with gratitude to the author for opening our mind to the pervading mental health challenges around us. I warmly commend Dr. Dwamena-Aboagye on her determination to complete the research and for the courage to share her findings with the rest of us.

—Allison M Howell
Associate Professor and Adjunct Staff, Akrofi-Christaller Institute of Theology, Mission and Culture
March 2021

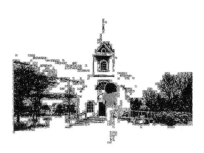

In this fascinating book, Dr. Angela Dwamena-Aboagye takes us on a pilgrimage through unchartered paths and examines 'what informs pastoral response to mental health and women's mental health problems.' The study is significant in all respects because the findings reveal the theological presuppositions and cultural biases that underlie the approaches used by pastoral care givers in dealing with issues that affect women's mental health and wellbeing; it makes a contribution to the nexus between science and the Christian faith and recommends ways by which policy makers, stake holders and care givers can cooperate in dealing with mental health issues. The book is a treasure trove, the reason why it must be read.

—Phillip Laryea, PhD
—*Associate Professor of African Theology and Dean of Accredited Studies, Akrofi-Christaller Institute, Ghana*

The published literature on mental health in Africa is not much and that of women, in particular, is even less. Angela's book fills an important niche in this knowledge gap. Of immense interest are the stories and perceptions of the brave and resilient women survivors who were willing to share their experiences of living with mental health challenges. They reveal systems of help that often failed them whether it was that of orthodox medicine, traditional or faith-based treatments.

From what the women said and from the pastors' interviews, the problem seems to be the tendency for pastors to consider the complexity of mental health challenges from the restricted viewpoint of spiritual disruption. As Angela points out, this is tunnel vision and pastors need to augment their knowledge of human functioning and team up with other mental health professionals to ensure holistic care for those who seek help. If pastors who read this book are motivated to get help to do this, the vision for this book would have been realized. It is also hoped that women with mental health challenges who read this book will be encouraged by the strength and resilience of the women who shared their experiences.

—Dr. Araba Sefa Dedeh
Clinical Psychologist and Senior Lecturer (Rtd), Dept of Psychiatry, University of Ghana School of Medicine and Dentistry
March 2021

While engaging mental health can be a taboo topic for some scholars, particularly in Africa, Dr. Angela Dwamena-Aboagye does not shy away from the subject but rather invites us to explore the interrelatedness of gender, culture, mental illness, and spirituality with indepth critical analyses. With lucidness and empathy, she details the plight of Ghanaian evangelical Christian women struggling to access care for mental health disruptions. Her overarching arguments surrounding the over-spiritualisation of mental illness, alongside of the risks of insufficient insight/training in mental health, therapeutic counselling, and bio-cultural influences upon female well-being are very well made, deserving urgent attention from church leaders, policy makers, academics, carers, and health workers in Africa. Equally, for Western scholars and international NGOs wishing to engage this important, underexplored topic, Dr. Dwamena-Aboagye has produced a scholarly and practical resource. Her convincing case for the benefits of a bio-psycho-socio-cultural-spiritual model of care encourages and invites dialogue and mutual learning between Africa and the West. I warmly recommend this accessible and insightful work.

—Dr. Sara Fretheim
University of Münster
March 2021

PREFACE

This book is one of two books I intend to publish from my doctoral thesis, completed in 2018 at Akrofi-Christaller Institute for Theology, Mission and Culture, Akropong-Akuapem, Ghana. The long title of my thesis is "Ministering to Hurting Women: An Analysis of the Cultural and Theological Understanding and Responses of Evangelical Ghanaian Pastors Regarding Women's Mental Health."

Indeed, this book is constituted from the second part of the thesis, which examines the perspectives of Ghanaian African Christian women of their first hand experiences with mental distress and illness and their interactions with Ghanaian Pastors in their attempt to seek help. This part of the study also delves into the minds of Ghanaian Pastors who belong to churches described as evangelical, as they attempt to provide help and support to people, including women who suffer emotional and mental distress and illnesses in their congregations, or those who approach them for assistance.

Hopefully, the second book will follow suit, God willing, soon. The second book will broadly examine the relationship between Christian Faith, Culture, Theology and Mental Health, addressed in the first part of my doctoral thesis. The questions raised by Christian sufferers over the ages, and the attempts to discern the mind of Christ and make meaning of these questions from a place of faith should continue to engage the minds of sufferers, ordinary people, scientists and scholars alike towards a worthy goal - the healing and restoration of loved ones and friends with mental health challenges.

CONTENTS

DEDICATION	iii
ACKNOWLEDGMENTS	iv
FOREWORD	vi
PREFACE	x
LIST OF ABBREVIATIONS	xv
LISTS OF TABLES	xv
CHAPTER ONE	1
WHY I CHOSE TO STUDY WOMEN'S MENTAL HEALTH	
AND PASTORAL RESPONSE IN GHANA	1
CHAPTER TWO	6
DEFINITIONS OF KEY TERMINOLOGY	6
Evangelical Christian	6
Evangelical Ghanaian Pastor	6
Health	7
Mental Health	7
Emotional Distresses, Mental Illness and Disorders	7
Women's Mental Health	9
Gender and Gender Relations	9
Theology	10
Culture	10
Primal	11
CHAPTER THREE	12
WOMEN, GENDER AND MENTAL HEALTH: A GLOBAL OVERVIEW	12
Men, Women and Mental Health	12
Social and Cultural Factors	14
Violence Against Women, Sexual and Gender-Based	
Violence (VAW/SGBV) and Women's Mental Health	16
Economic Factors	17
Biological and Neurological Factors	17
Intersectionalities	18
Gendered Social Responses	19
Help-seeking Behaviour	19
Treatment Response	20
CHAPTER FOUR	21
HOW CHRISTIAN WOMEN COPE WITH MENTAL	
HEALTH CHALLENGES AND THE ROLE OF THE CHURCH	21
PASTORAL ROLE IN EMOTIONAL AND MENTAL HEALTH	
RESPONSE	24

CHAPTER FIVE   27
OVERVIEW OF MENTAL HEALTH IN GHANA   27
General Mental Health Data   27
Public Facilities and Services   28
Alternative Care and Issues Arising   28
Socio-cultural Issues, Stigma and Social Responses   29
Policy and Legislative Issues   30
ADVOCACY AND MOBILISATION FOR PROMOTING
MENTAL HEALTH ISSUES   31
SOME WOMEN'S HEALTH ISSUES THAT IMPINGE ON
WOMEN'S MENTAL HEALTH IN GHANA   32
Maternal Mortality   32
Violence against Women in Ghana   33
Women's Disability Status   34
WOMEN'S MENTAL HEALTH IN GHANA   34
Perceptions about Ghanaian Women with Mental and
Emotional Distress   35
A Note on Depression (and other Mental Disorders) in
Ghanaian Women and the Connection with Witchcraft   36
CHAPTER SIX   40
GHANAIAN CHRISTIAN WOMEN'S EXPERIENCES OF MENTAL
HEALTH CHALLENGES AND THEIR PERSPECTIVES ON RESPONSES 40
Introduction   40
Perceptions of Causes of Respondents' Emotional/Mental Ill-health   42
Manifesting Symptoms   46
Perceived Connection between Mental Illness and Femaleness   48
Societal Attitudes and Responses to their Condition of Mental Illness 49
Seeking Help   50
Experiences with Specific Pastoral Responses from EGPs   57
Collaboration between EGPs and Professional Mental Health
Practitioners   58
Perception of the Knowledge base of EGPs   59
Recommendations for EGPs and Churches   60
Personal Faith and Spirituality and Coping with Emotional/
Mental Distress   61
CHAPTER SEVEN   64
PASTORS RESPONDING: PERCEPTIONS ON SYMPTOMS,
GENDER DIFFERENCES AND CAUSES   64
Introduction   64
Evangelical Ghanaian Pastors' (EGPs) Views and Perceptions on

Symptoms, Gender Differences and Causes of Emotional or
Mental Distress and Illness   66
Summary and Conclusion   83
CHAPTER EIGHT   84
PASTORS RESPONDING: INTERVENTIONS,
KNOWLEDGE, COLLABOARATION, THEOLOGICAL AND
CULTURAL UNDERSTANDING   84
Introduction   84
Pastoral Responses (or Practical Interventions) to Address Cases of
Emotional/Mental Distress and Illness   84
EGPs' Knowledge base of Abnormal Psychology/Mental Illness   96
EGPs' cultural perceptions and understanding of emotional
distress and mental illness   103
Theological Perspectives of EGPs on Mental Health and Mental
Distress/Illness   110
Support of EGPs and Evangelical Churches (E-Churches) for
Women's Roles and for Women in Distress   119
EGPs' Perspectives on How Evangelical Ghanaian Churches
Must Respond   122
EGPs' Perspectives on Formal Collaboration with Professional
Mental Health Practitioners   125
CHAPTER NINE   129
A CALL TO 'DO JUSTICE AND SHOW MERCY'   129
Introduction   129
Discussion of Findings and Implications   130
REFLECTIONS   133
EGPs cannot Recognise and Respond to Women's Mental
Health Issues without Understanding Mental Health Generally   133
The Story of Two Women: Trusting that God is in the Process of Cure,
Healing and Wholeness   134
Over-spiritualisation, Over-medicalisation and EGPs'
Potential Role and Relevant Ministry in an African Context   136
The Bio-Psycho-Socio-Cultural-Spiritual Model: Adopting and
Adapting a Framework for Ministry   139
The Leadership Role of Christian Faith and Theology in Adopting
an Integrated Model of Understanding and Response   142
Gender-sensitivity in a Ministry to Hurting Women   144
SIGNIFICANT RECOMMENDATIONS FROM RESPONDENTS   145
MY RECOMMENDATIONS   146
Government of Ghana   146

Mental Health Professionals   147
Caregivers   148
The Distressed/Sufferer   148
Christian Women   149
EGPs and their Churches   150
CONCLUSION   152
BIBLIOGRAPHY   185

LIST OF ABBREVIATIONS

AEA	Association of Evangelicals in Africa
AIC	African Independent/Initiated Church
APA	American Psychiatric Association
ATR	African Traditional Religion
AOG	Assemblies of God
COP	Church of Pentecost
DSM	Diagnostic Statistical Manual (of the APA)
DOVVSU	Domestic Violence and Victims' Support Unit
EGP	Evangelical Ghanaian Pastor
GOG	Government of Ghana
GLSS	Ghana Living Standards Survey
GSS	Ghana Statistical Service
ICD	International Classification of Diseases (of WHO)
ICGC	International Central Gospel Church
MDGs	Millennium Development Goals
MHA	Mental Health Authority
MHP	Mental Health Professional
MoGSCP	Ministry of Gender, Children and Social Protection
MOH	Ministry of Health
NDPC	National Development Planning Commission
OCD	Obsessive Compulsion Disorder
PCG	Presbyterian Church of Ghana
SGBV	Sexual and Gender-Based Violence
UGMS	University of Ghana Medical School
VAW	Violence Against Women
WHO	World Health Organization

LISTS OF TABLES

Table 1	Profile of Christian Women Survivors of Emotional/Mental Illness Interviewed
Table 2	Profile of Evangelical Ghanaian Pastors (EGP) Respondents

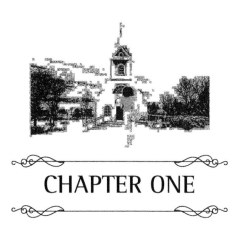

CHAPTER ONE

WHY I CHOSE TO STUDY WOMEN'S MENTAL HEALTH AND PASTORAL RESPONSE IN GHANA

Pastors of the evangelical tradition in Ghana, as heads of their local churches and denominations, are involved in various leadership, administrative and shepherding activities. Shepherding or caring for the flock is seen as central to their calling, particularly in the context of ministering in economically depressed communities compounded by increasing social vices and socio-political inequalities.

The available literature suggests that pastoral care (and counselling), which also involves assisting congregants to handle emotional and psychological problems, is highly valued in many Christian communities around the world. There is however a dearth of research on how pastors in Ghana, particularly evangelical pastors, understand the nature of mental health issues, especially as they affect women, who are the majority in their congregations. It is difficult to know their cultural and theological perceptions about mental health issues; nor is it easy to discern how they relate such perceptions or understanding to their specific pastoral responses to people facing emotional distress or psychological problems.

I chose this area of study for a number of personal and professional reasons. First, I am an evangelical Ghanaian Christian woman, who is a member of a Pentecostal-Charismatic congregation and a mental illness survivor. In 2008, I was diagnosed with severe Obsessive Compulsive Disorder (OCD) and depression. For more than three years, I went through what could be described as the 'dark night of the soul' experience. Although my church family and pastors provided much support and kindness, I recognise that the extent of their understanding of my suffering influenced the nature of their responses to my distress. I found that almost all the pastors who tried to help me in my plight really had no notion about the nature of my particular symptoms; yet, they purported to counsel me, while others took me through prayer and deliverance sessions.

I also have Christian women friends and acquaintances who have suffered or survived mental distress and illness. They, too, have stories of their experiences and challenges, as well as the response of church leaders and the church community to their issues. As a fellow survivor, I identify with these friends, some of whom were specifically selected to participate in this study.

Also, I have worked in the area of advocacy and empowerment of women for more than two decades. Part of my professional work has been to provide direct support to female survivors of sexual, domestic and other gender-based abuses in Ghana, many of whom are Christians. I have had to confront mental health problems in those who have faced such abuses, such as low self-esteem, flashbacks, hyper-vigilance, anxiety, depression, paranoia and other serious psychological effects and disorders. Working alongside others, including social workers, professional psychologists, psychiatrists and clergy, I have given these women and girls the necessary assistance within my professional mandate, in spite of the restrictive context within which I work.[1]

Operating within such a context, I have recognised that Christians, particularly Ghanaian Christian women, invariably turn first to their pastors (as I did) when experiencing any form of emotional or mental distress, or inexplicable life challenges. Since pastors are considered an important resource in such situations, it became a subject of interest for me to explore in depth, first, the evangelical pastor's understanding of mental health and, in particular, women's mental health issues; and, second, why pastors appear to choose certain modes or actions as their first-line responses to such problems. Similarly, in a context where mental illness is stigmatised and any discussion on it is still largely viewed as taboo, my interest in Christian women's experience of mental illness and how they seek help is of particular importance. This is because any research or advocacy actions that lead to improved services and support for women in such situations, ultimately add to the general improvement of the welfare and rights of women and to the betterment of the general population in Ghana.

The fundamental presupposition of this study was that, by their numbers, women dominate in the evangelical churches in Ghana. For them, the church is more than an assembly of believers and a place of worship. It is a community to belong to, a safe haven where one seeks and obtains help from God, one's pastor and the family of believers in times of distress or trouble. When Ghanaian Christian women have problems (including mental illness or emotional distress) and personal coping strategies fail, they are most likely to seek help from their pastors in the first instance. In situations of emotional or mental distress or illness, pastors are expected to show empathy and engage in a range of pastoral care activities to help restore the sufferer to normalcy. The presumption therefore is that Christian women who are appropriately supported and assisted by their pastors are more likely to manage their symptoms and recover or heal much better than those who are not given such appropriate support. Thus, a pastor's response to a woman's mental health problem (or any other person for that matter) may either help mitigate the problem or cause more harm. In other words, evangelical Ghanaian pastors who are able to recognise and understand the emotional and mental problems of the women in their congregations and respond with appropriate pastoral care approaches, are likely to get better or more effective results from their actions. This could lead to a better management of the symptoms of distress, recovery and even healing for the women. The question, then, is this: what comprises 'appropriate pastoral care approaches' for Ghanaian evangelical pastors ministering to hurting people, in particular, women?

It has been a concern that advances in Western scientific enquiry and epistemology in the medical and psychological fields have led to therapeutic approaches that have influenced the manner in which persons with mental issues have been cared for. These advances have, to some degree, also influenced pastoral care approaches and practices in the Western Church. With the influence of scientific rationality, Western approaches to psychological disorders have tended towards more medicalisation and psychotherapy practices that until recently paid little attention to the spiritual experiences of mental illness sufferers. Modern psychology's relationship to religion, theology and the Christian faith in particular has been found to be largely tenuous and fractious.[2] However, in the last few decades, Christian scholars and practitioners in the field of psychology have expended significant effort to retrieve the Christian tradition which views human beings not merely as physical beings, but as beings with components of spirit, soul and body. This is to ensure that Christians working in the mental health arena, whether as lay persons, clergy or professional therapists and counsellors, adopt and use approaches that best respond to the 'whole' of the human experience with mental distress and ill-health.

On the other hand, African Christians appear not to have much difficulty understanding human beings as comprising spirit, soul and body. This study is based thus on the premise that in Ghana, mental health sufferers, their families, communities and persons who purport to help them recover whether clergy, lay people or professional therapists all live in this worldview and share its basic belief in the existence of the spiritual world. At the very least, these helpers or caregivers contend on a daily basis with people who believe in the *primal* spiritual world.[3]

Indeed, I found through this study that the African cultural and spiritual worldview influences evangelical Ghanaian pastors' understanding of and response to mental health issues among their congregants, especially women; that it is perhaps this cultural and theological understanding of mental health problems which leads evangelical Ghanaian pastors to over-spiritualise mental health issues. The term, *Over-spiritualisation*, connotes the view that symptoms or disturbances are primarily or solely caused by spiritual factors such as demonic possession, demonic oppression or attack; being cursed by an offended person; the result of one's sinfulness or sinful behaviour; being under an ancestral or family generational curse and other such related causes. Consequently, a pastor's over-spiritualisation of mental or emotional disturbances may invariably lead to the employment of spiritual actions and strategies being prescribed for the sufferer in the form of engagement in intense and long prayers, fasting, deliverance sessions (in other literature referred to as *exorcism,* even though some theologians distinguish between the two), or sending the patient to a prayer or healing camp where these regimens are expected to be undertaken.

Thus it was necessary to examine what informs pastoral response to mental health and women's mental health problems, and to examine in depth the theological and cultural assumptions and worldviews that underlie their choice of response. Women's voices needed to be heard in this quest-Ghanaian evangelical Christian women who have experienced both mental illness and the pastoral response or assistance they received. It was also important to hear the voices of the all-important pastoral responders and to understand the perspectives and basis of their practices. What I gathered is what I share in this book.

It is note-worthy that interest in mental health has grown exponentially world-wide in the last decade. In Ghana, it has been quite startling to see mental health, a culturally taboo subject for many families at the time I started my doctoral research in 2013, become more and more demystified as at the time I was reviewing this work for publication. There are now so many more organizations, coalitions, networks, online programs and webinars in Ghana addressing mental health from myriad perspectives. This increasing interest has been given greater impetus by the COVID-19 pandemic which took the world by storm in the year 2020 and continues to intrigue many scientists and medical practitioners due to the neurological and psychological impacts the disease appears to be spurning on some of its victims. Many of these efforts at addressing mental health issues, however, remain in the professionalized realm of science spearheaded primarily by mental health practitioners such as psychiatrists, psychologists and psychiatric nurses. The publication of this study thus attempts to bring on board the critical role of a group of apparent first line responders to sufferers, being Pastors, simply because of who we are as Africans a notoriously religious people who would prefer to seek a solution from God first and if Christians, mostly through the agency of the Pastor, before consulting anything or anybody else.

It is hoped that this work contributes to the broader vision of improving the welfare and condition of people generally and also in particular women, as valuable and vital members of the Ghanaian Church. There is also the hope that this work garners more support for greater collaboration between science and the Christian faith, as well as the seeking of the mind of God in the attempt to provide answers to one of life's most puzzling questions -mental illness. For after all, Jesus Christ is still the Lord who heals His people (Exodus 15:26); He is Lord over everything (Philippians 2:11), and by Him all things consist and hold together (Col 1:17).

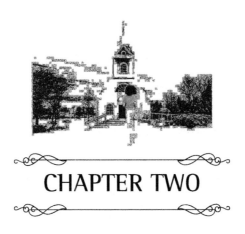

CHAPTER TWO

DEFINITIONS OF KEY TERMINOLOGY

Evangelical Christian

Evangelical Christians are generally those who believe the Bible is the authoritative and inspired Word of God.[4] They believe in the Triune God, the deity of Jesus Christ and the personal repentance and acceptance by an individual of His substitutionary death as the only means by which one's sinfulness can be atoned for, in order to gain salvation and reconciliation with God. Evangelicals are united in their belief about the regenerating work of the Holy Spirit and His empowerment for godly living. Evangelicals believe in the spiritual unity of all who believe in Jesus Christ as Saviour and Lord. The point must be made that unlike the practice in Western Christianity where there are sharp distinctions made between churches considered evangelical and those that are not, in the generality of the African Church, the claim to the evangelical tradition is not so clear cut; as long as a Christian denomination or believer predominantly shares in the evangelical views of Christianity, they are evangelical – be they Methodists, Presbyterians, Baptists, Anglicans, Episcopalians, Pentecostal, or Charismatic, including Catholic Charismatics.[5]

Evangelical Ghanaian Pastor

An evangelical Ghanaian Pastor (EGP) therefore, is a pastor of a recognized church denomination that identifies itself with the evangelical tradition. The Presbyterian Church of Ghana, Assemblies of God (Ghana), Church of Pentecost and the International Central Gospel Church, whose pastors were the participants of this study all identify themselves as evangelical.

Health

Health is defined as "a state of complete physical, mental, and social well-being and not merely the absence of disease or infirmity."[6] Toews writes that "health is more than the absence of disease... it is a positive state of well-being." [7] A human being's state of health comprises physical, psychological, social, economic, political, environmental and spiritual aspects all aspects interacting to make the human being wholly healthy.

Mental Health

Although mental illness is difficult to define,[8] some definitions have been proffered by institutions and individuals, mainly professional. In 2001 WHO defined "mental health" as "...a state of well-being in which the individual realizes his or her abilities, can cope with the normal stresses of life, can work productively and fruitfully, and is able to make a contribution to his or her community."[9] The American Psychiatric Association (APA) defines mental disorder as "a clinically significant behavioral or psychological syndrome or pattern that occurs in a person and that is associated with present distress (a painful syndrome) or disability (impairment in one or more important areas of functioning) or with a significantly increased risk of suffering death, pain, disability, or an important loss of freedom."[10] In the book *Where There Is No Psychiatrist*, written by Vikram Patel for health workers in developing countries, mental illness is "any illness experienced by a person which affects their emotions, thoughts or behavior, which is out of keeping with their cultural beliefs and personality, and is producing a negative effect on their lives or the lives of their families".[11]

Emotional Distresses, Mental Illness and Disorders

In popular usage, emotional or mental distress, mental ill-health, mental illness and mental disorders are often used interchangeably. In the literature I reviewed, I also found some scholarly attempts to bring some understanding on the distinctions between emotional problems (or distress) and mental illness. One such attempt is from Harold Koenig who writes: "By emotional problems, I mean short or long-term struggles with depression, anxiety, or other difficulties with mood or happiness. By mental illness, I mean schizophrenia, bi-polar disorder and other long-term psychoses or other personality disorders."[12] For mental illness, Stanford, a neuro-psychiatrist defines it as: "... a disorder of the brain resulting in the disruption of a person's thoughts, feelings, moods, and ability to relate to others that is severe enough to require psychological or psychiatric intervention... A mental illness... is a debilitating experience in which the person is simply unable to function normally for an extended period of time."[13]

However, the formal categorizations of mental ill-health conditions from both the World Health Organization (WHO) and the American Psychiatric Association (APA) seem not to make such distinctions between emotional distresses and mental illness, as all known and classified emotional or mental-related conditions which cause distress (affecting the psyche) are deemed conditions of mental ill-health.

In effect, for human beings, there may be a continuum from having minor emotional or mental problems, challenges or distresses which may arise out of life's issues or crises to a state of having a serious or major mental condition with psychotic features.[14] For example, one may be in a state of not being able to sleep well (insomnia) for a few weeks due to concerns about a truant child. This is seen as experiencing some form of mental ill-health arising out of a stressful situation; however, if one continues to experience lack of sleep over a much longer period affecting ability to function normally, then a more serious mental ill-health problem may be developing. Again, many of the conditions classified as 'phobias' are often seen as minor mental ill-health conditions,[15] while those with psychotic features such as 'schizophrenia' are deemed major. It is part of the practice of mental health professionals, such as clinical psychologists or psychiatrists, to diagnose if a serious mental illness condition is present in an individual or not.

It is important to note however, that it is not always the case that an emotionally or mentally disturbing situation arising out of life's crises carries an automatic risk of developing into a serious mental illness condition or disorder. However, it is also true that an unmanaged distress from a life crisis situation may degenerate into a serious mental health condition, for example, unmanaged grief from the loss of a loved one could degenerate into major depression.

It is also possible to have the ability to deal with life's issues constructively, even when one is experiencing a diagnosed mental disorder. Much depends on how a particular situation or condition is being experienced by the sufferer.[16]

There are two formally accepted internationally recognized classifications of mental illnesses or disorders.[17] The first is the APA's *Diagnostic and Statistical Manual* (DSM) which has gone through five revisions since 1952, the latest named DSM-5.[18] There is also the International Classification of Diseases (ICD) from the World Health Organization (WHO), which has had ten revisions since 1948.[19] From the formal classifications, there are several known or accepted mental conditions or disorders. With scientific advancement, new disorders are constantly being discovered, classified or re-classified.[20] Broadly, mental disorders fall under the following categories: Anxiety and related disorders (e.g., Generalized Anxiety Disorder); Mood disorders (e.g., Depression); Psychotic disorders (e.g., Schizophrenia); Brain Injury or Disease disorders (e.g., Dementia and Mental Retardation conditions); Trauma related disorders (e.g., Post-Traumatic Stress Disorder); and Substance Abuse disorders (e.g., Alcohol and Narcotic abuse disorders). Others are Sleep disorders; Sexual disorders; Maladaptive Personality Disorders (e.g., Borderline Personality disorder); and Childhood related disorders (e.g., Attention Deficit Hyperactive Disorder).[21]

Vikram Patel adds an important cultural dimension to how mental illness should be viewed. He asserts:

It is of great importance...to recognise that the term 'mental illness' does not refer to a homogeneous group of problems, but rather to a number of different types of disorder. It is even more important to recognise that, although every society has people it views as mentally ill, the use and construction of this concept may vary considerably from one society to another.[22]

Women's Mental Health

Susan G. Kornstein and Anita H. Clayton describe women's health as including "health issues and diseases that are unique to women, such as gynaecological conditions; diseases that are more prevalent in women; and diseases that are expressed differently in women and men."[23] In the same vein, women's mental health can be said to be those conditions in women pertaining to their mental health, which may be unique to women because of their sex. It also entails psychological conditions more prevalent in women compared to men, as well as mental conditions which are expressed differently in women and men. This description implies that women may present with different symptoms, have a more serious form of a particular condition, or have a different course of an illness, or respond differently to interventions for treatment or care.[24]

Gender and Gender Relations

Basically, the term gender describes '...those characteristics of men and women which are *socially* determined, in contrast to those which are *biologically* determined.'[25] Although gender relations are about how men and women *relate to each other* within the parameters of their roles and expected social behaviours, it also refers to *inequality* in relations between men and women acquired in the process of socialisation. This is depicted in the roles of men and women in power sharing, decision-making, division of labour and returns from labour at all levels, including household and community levels.[26]

Theology

The root meaning of theology is "the study of God."[27] Kwame Bediako taught that theology is an attempt to say something about God, in the belief that God has already said something about Himself and His dealings, purposes and relationship with humankind and His creation.[28] Andrew Walls also gives a simple but profound understanding of the purpose of (Christian) theology; that is, "to make or clarify Christian decisions". He wrote that theology: "... is about choices... an attempt to think in a Christian way. And the need for choice and decision arises from specific settings in life."[29] In this study, pastoral understanding of and response to women's mental health issues, issues that arise from culture-specific contexts and worldviews interacting with the Christian religion and faith are thought through and analysed from the point of seeking Christian answers to puzzling questions of life–theologically.

Culture

The term "culture" has several definitions with common features. Bediako stresses the importance of culture in shaping people's identity, thought and actions, referring to its dimensions as "language, arts, crafts, eating habits, patterns of social relationships, how men, women and children relate, how they ought to relate, how they see each other."[30] He also adds that "Political organization, notions of leadership, authority, power and rule are also dimensions of culture. Religious and moral values, things deemed acceptable and unacceptable are all elements of culture"[31]

Mental health issues occur within cultural contexts. Culture has an impact on how mental distress or illness is perceived and treated. One description of culture I deem particularly relevant to this subject is as follows:

> Culture provides meaning to social interactions through a pervasive set of symbols that are reciprocally built up out of everyday experiences of social life. *Through all these elements, culture patterns ways of thinking, feeling and reacting.* Consequently, culture shapes and guides the behaviours and the expectations of individuals. *Cultural rules govern the expression of emotion and the expectations regarding the role of the individual in society.*[32]

In sum, aspects of culture include language, meanings, knowledge, beliefs, rules and norms, values and religion and these in turn shape expectations of society regarding behavior and even expression of emotion.[33] Eshun, et al., observe:

> [C]ulture has been conceptualized as something that is learned, changes over time, is cyclical or self-reinforcing, consists of tangible and intangible behaviors, and most important of all, is crucial for survival and adaptation. *Cultural traits and norms do influence how we think, how we respond to distress, and how comfortable we are expressing our emotions.*[34]

Despite having enduring features, culture however is not static; it is dynamic, constantly evolving, and subject to various influences, particularly contact with other cultures and cultural movements.[35] Within culture, there is a "continual interplay resulting in dynamism, adaptability, re-interpretation, re-formulation and change."[36]

Primal

The term 'primal' according to Andrew Walls, is used to describe the "... religions of the circumpolar peoples of various peoples of Africa, the Indian sub-continent, South East Asia, Inner Asia, North and South America, Australia and the Pacific... Primal is not a euphemism for "primitive"... The word helpfully underlines two features of the religions of the peoples indicated: their historical anteriority and their basic elemental status in human experience."[37] G. M Bediako explains that: "Primal means...universal basic elements of human understanding of the Transcendent and the world, essential and valid religious insights that may be built upon or suppressed, but not superseded."[38]

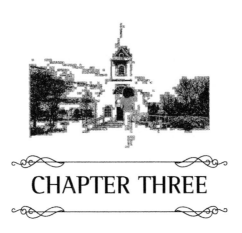

CHAPTER THREE

WOMEN, GENDER AND MENTAL HEALTH :
A GLOBAL OVERVIEW

Men, Women and Mental Health

As explained earlier, women's mental health are conditions in women pertaining to their mental health, and conditions which may be unique to women because of their sex.[1] There are psychological conditions more prevalent in women than men, as well as conditions expressed and experienced differently in women and men.[2] Women therefore may present with different symptoms, have a more serious form of a particular condition, have a different course of an illness, or respond differently to interventions for treatment or care.[3] Many scholars have pointed out that women are exposed to mental distress and illness sometimes just by reason of their sex or being female. Thus, post-partum depression, for example, affects only females because they give birth to children. Women may also be susceptible as a result of gendered expectations, such as the distress resulting from the perceived inability to fulfil multiple roles as expected by their families, society or themselves. Sex and gender issues are therefore important in the global discussion on women's mental health for creating awareness, determining causality, providing care and treatment, as well as in policy-making.

With reference to health, gender 'influences the control men and women have over the determinants of their health, for example, their economic position and social status, and their access to resources... Gender is a powerful social determinant of health that interacts with other variables such as age, family structure, income, education and social support, and with a variety of behavioral factors.'[4] Vikram Patel explains the importance of sex and gender in health:

Sex and gender are both important determinants of health. Biological sex and socially-constructed gender interact to produce differential risks and vulnerability to ill health, and differences in health-seeking behavior and health outcomes for women and men.[5]

In relation to mental health specifically, Nancy Musinguzi notes that

Gender plays a significant role in understanding mental health as a vital issue in global affairs. Gender establishes the dynamics of power and control the sexes hold over socioeconomic factions of their personal lives, social status, accessibility to treatment in their respective societies, and their vulnerability to particular mental health risks.[6]

Lauren Slater argues that taking a sex and gender-based approach to mental health can be beneficial to both men and women, including understanding more about what causes mental health problems at different times in a person's life.[7] This is important, she posits, because men and women are different 'in mind and body, in soma and psyche'.[8] Men and women are also different 'in hormonal development, in brain development, in physiological development, and in social development'.[9]

Susan G. Kornstein and Anita H. Clayton point out that 'interest in women's health has grown' in the West only in the last few decades.[10] They further add that

Until recently, women were excluded from clinical trials... what was learned from studies of men was presumed to carry over to women. Moreover, in the studies that included women, the data usually were not analyzed separately by gender... We are now learning that there are important gender differences to consider in both assessment and treatment. We are learning that some diseases show different symptoms, a different course of illness, and/or different risk factors in men and women.[11]

D.E. Stewart and his co-authors also confirm that women have the same overall prevalence of psychiatric disorders as men, but most countries show differences in diagnosis by sex.[12] Also, there are considerable differences globally in the sex ratios for selected mental disorders, with women having much higher rates for disorders such as major depression, anxiety disorders, posttraumatic stress disorder, and eating disorders.[13] Alcohol and drug abuse are reportedly less prevalent in women than men globally, but still present a significant mental health problem for many women.[14]

Differences also exist in epidemiology, risk factors, presentation of symptoms, course of illness, co-morbidity and treatment response.[15] Thus, for example, although bipolar disorder is almost equally prevalent in the sexes, women tend to have more rapid mood cycling.[16] With schizophrenia,

Vivian K. Burt and Victoria C. Hendrick report that the course of this disorder is less severe in women, who tend to have a later onset of it in life, fewer symptoms and better treatment response than men.[17] In the United States, for example, women are four times more likely than men to attempt suicide, though less likely to die from the attempt.[18] However, men have much higher rates of suicide compared to women across the world.[19] Eating disorders such as anorexia and bulimia nervosa are more common with women because of media promotion of 'the cult of thinness' as the ideal body image for women, particularly in the West.[20]Research also shows that gender differences in patterns of mental distress vary, depending on one's phase in life from childhood, through adolescence into adulthood.[21]

Social and Cultural Factors

Socio-cultural factors and psychosocial determinants also significantly demonstrate how women and men become vulnerable or respond to mental distress or illness differently.[22] Stewart and his co-authors stress that

> Women's life experiences differ from those of men in many ways, including child bearing and rearing, women's double shifts (at home and at work) and their lack of power in personal, working, economic, social and professional relationships... [t]hese experiences have an impact on women's self-esteem, sense of mastery, and mood.[23]

The multiple roles women juggle feature significantly in many articles on women's mental health. For example, Angela Barron McBride in her investigation asserts that

> [M]ultiple roles are associated with competing demands, which can lead to role overload and resulting strain. Measures of the role strain include somatization, depression, anxiety-obsessive compulsiveness, discomfort, anger/hostility, and dissatisfaction.[24]

Multiple roles include women's marital and parenting roles, household responsibilities such as cleaning, cooking, shopping, as well as holding part-time or full-time formal jobs. Increasingly across the globe, many women are also providing care for elderly parents and sometimes for in-laws.[25] Burt and Hendrick also report that with women,

> [M]any face daily challenges to fulfill multiple roles and meet conflicting demands. Furthermore, women's traditionally disadvantaged social status, lower wages, and increased vulnerability to sexual and domestic violence may contribute to their higher rates of depressive and anxiety disorders.[26]

On their part, Kornstein and Clayton insist that

Gender differences in socialization processes and rates of traumatic abuse, as well as the various social roles of women as wives, mothers, caretakers of elderly parents, and workers, all deserve consideration in understanding risk factors for mental illness and the effects of these disorders on women and their families.[27]

Interestingly, being a woman in a Western or non-Western culture may enhance or undermine mental health, depending on certain factors. Nalini Pandalangat makes the following observation:

Collectivistic or primarily non-Western cultures require a high level of relatedness and moderate levels of autonomy to maintain mental health...Many developing nations have collectivistic cultures, which have greater connectedness than Western cultures and extensive social networks. Hence in social contexts where there is a moderate level of autonomy, a woman's degree of social and emotional connectedness, by virtue of her gender role as a caregiver, mother and nurturer might actually enhance her mental wellbeing...However, where the cultural context in developing countries or within communities stresses the caregiving and homemaker roles while devaluing the contribution of women and disempowering them, then this is a ready formula for mental health problems.[28]

Societal gender discrimination and higher vulnerability to factors such as child prostitution, human trafficking and sexual tourism have all been cited as important considerations affecting women's mental health.[29] Also, where there are mental health problems in a family, the burden of care usually falls on women.[30] In her study, Husna Razee found that with women in the Maldives, adverse life circumstances, including entrapment and humiliation within marriage, facing desertion by a husband, being left with several children to care for and severe socio-economic difficulties without adequate safety nets contributed to women's mental distress.[31]

Other significant social factors impinge on women's mental health globally. Of significance are the lack of equal access to education and the lack of quality reproductive health services.[32] Women's infertility and its cultural implications and women's vulnerability to certain infectious diseases such as HIV/AIDS also affect women's mental health.[33] Civil conflicts and environmental disasters have equally marked effects on women's mental health, especially regarding the caregiving roles they are expected to play during and in the aftermath of such occurrences.[34]

Violence Against Women, Sexual and Gender-Based Violence (VAW/SGBV) and Women's Mental Health

Violence against women (VAW) and sexual and gender-based violence (SGBV), which globally affect women and girls in higher numbers than men and boys, generally have their roots in patriarchal notions and societal perceptions of women's inferior social positioning.[35] No doubt, VAW and SGBV have a profound negative impact on women's mental health wherever the phenomena occur. VAW and SGBV involve acts of coercion, control, intimidation and humiliation encompassing physical, psychological/emotional, sexual and economic forms of abusive conduct, within or outside the domestic sphere.

Specific forms of VAW and SGBV include assault and battery, rape and sexual harassment, threats and insulting behaviour, destruction of economic means or property, enforced isolation, as well as trafficking and forced prostitution, among others. VAW and SGBV also encompass various forms of harmful traditional or cultural practices in parts of the world, such as dehumanising widowhood and puberty rites, witchcraft accusation, female genital mutilation/cutting, female customary servitude and others.[36] The resulting impact of such acts on the victimised includes fear, anxiety, loss of control, low self-esteem and other conditions linked with mental disorders.[37] Astbury's reports are insightful:

> Gender-based violence in childhood and adult life, including physical, sexual and emotional violence and abuse, is associated with threefold to fourfold increase in risk of depression and is also linked with marked increases in psychiatric comorbidity, including increased rates of anxiety, post-traumatic stress disorder, suicidality, substance abuse disorders, somatization, panic disorders, eating disorders, and certain personality disorders such as borderline personality disorder.[38]

The WHO also indicates that

> The high prevalence of sexual violence to which women are exposed and the correspondingly high rate of Post Traumatic Stress Disorder (PTSD) following such violence, renders women the largest single group of people affected by this disorder.[39]

There is no doubt, therefore, from the global data, that finding effective ways to prevent and address VAW and SGBV through all necessary legitimate means will have a significant impact in promoting mental health states globally.

Economic Factors

According to global statistics, women represent disproportionate percentages of the poor.[40] Women's poverty increases their dependence, undermines access to health and other social services for themselves and their families, as well as increasing their vulnerability to abuse and exploitation. Further important considerations are involved in addressing women's mental health.[41] They include economic difficulties faced by the increasing number of women who head households across the world and elderly women who tend to live longer than men and have increased risks of illnesses. There are also women deprived of their property and inheritance rights due to cultural beliefs and perceptions of the inferior status of women.

Biological and Neurological Factors

Gender differences in biological and neurological factors impinge on mental health for women and men. Thus, gender-related biological differences may also explain some of the notable differences between men and women's mental disorders. Research has revealed that women's brain anatomy is different from that of men. For example, the US Surgeon-General's Report of 2017 states that

> There are sex-based differences in the size and structure of the human brain. Men's brains are larger than women's. Women's brains are lighter but more complex, with proportionately larger frontal lobes (attributed to executive functions such as judgment, language, memory, problem solving, and socialization).[42]

Moreover, male and female reproductive hormones are known to produce different psychoactive effects in the sexes.[43] The reproductive events in women's lives equally play a major role in women's health, including mental health. Emotional stresses and mental disorders in women are reported to be common during childbearing years, while reproductive events act as triggers for the onset of mental illnesses or exacerbation of symptoms.[44] Women are prone to develop mental distress or illness symptoms during pre-menstrual, menopause or peri-menopausal stages. Post-partum illnesses such as depression, anxiety or OCDs are also reported in the female population globally.[45] Women who experience certain recurrent gynaecological conditions, such as genital warts or herpes, are affected negatively in sexual functioning and emotional wellbeing. Hysterectomies and other female related surgeries may also affect women's self-esteem and relationships with their partners.[46]

Furthermore, in countries where child marriages and teenage motherhood are highly prevalent, women's quality of life is adversely affected. These social issues in turn affect the maternal mortality rate, which is high in African and South Asian countries. High maternal mortality and child morbidity rates primarily occur because of poor access to quality healthcare, bad infrastructure, high fertility rates and the inferior status accorded women in socio-cultural belief systems.[47] All these factors contribute to the poor mental states of women.

Intersectionalities

Razee believes that it is necessary to explore women's individual life circumstances and how these affect their mental wellbeing, especially women in non-Western cultures.[48] This is because the majority of research studies on sex and gender differences in mental distress and illness have been drawn from Western sources. Besides, factors of race, status, age and availability of resources, among others, intersect mental wellbeing, In Ghana, for instance, V. de Menil, A. Osei and others point out in their study that the relationship between mental, physical and reproductive health in particular must be better understood.[49] They also stress that further investigation of the relationship between mental health and social determinants in Ghana is required.[50]

In mental health or illness, gender also intersects with social and protective factors deriving from race, ethnicity and culture. According to the US Surgeon-General's report,

> There is clearly much still to be learned about **social and protective factors** that affect mental health, including the effects of race, ethnicity, and culture... Rates of depression are higher among Hispanic and Caucasian women compared with African-American women. Similarly, there are considerable differences among women in rates of attempted suicide. Although women are more likely on average to attempt suicide than men, the rates of suicide attempts in African-American women are very low. These differences lead us to wonder if there are social or protective factors at play and underscore the fact that we need to understand more fully what happens with groups that do well.[51]

It would be interesting to investigate why there are much lower depression and suicide attempts in African-American women than in Hispanic and Caucasian women. Indeed, more research is required to determine whether this could be attributable to factors of differing historical, social or religious context among women of the afore-mentioned races.[52]

Gendered Social Responses

Societal responses to mental distress or illness depict gendered differences. It has been suggested that women with mental illnesses experience greater stigma and societal rejection than men.[53] The likelihood of a mentally ill man getting a marriage partner is higher than a mentally ill woman's chances.[54] In many societies, mentally ill women are sent out of their marital homes to their own relatives for care, while a mentally ill married man is expected to be primarily cared for by his wife.[55] Mental illness in women also has a more profound effect on family life in general because of the woman's role as the manager of the household.[56]

Help-seeking Behaviour

Some scholars suggest that men and women with mental health issues exhibit different patterns of help-seeking behaviour. In general, more women than men seek services for mental health problems within the primary care setting.[57] For instance, de Menil and his co-researchers assert that in Ghana, while men with disorders are perceived as a threat and are more likely to be taken to the psychiatric hospital for treatment, women with somatic complaints, on the other hand, seek treatment more commonly at churches, shrines and with primary care providers.[58] Other factors such as marital status influence help-seeking behaviour. In a study conducted by general practitioners (GPs) in Ireland, it was found that male respondents who were married or cohabiting were three times more likely to contact their GP for emotional problems than those who were single. It is possible that the support of their wives and partners mediated the men's willingness to seek help despite male-associated self-stigma.[59]

Differences in help-seeking behaviour also often depend on the particular problem. For example, Patel makes the point that for alcohol use disorders, both women and men rarely seek help, but for different reasons. While women are more likely to drink in secret because of the stigma associated with their drinking alcohol, men are less likely to see their drinking as a problem because of greater social acceptability of men using alcohol.[60] Similarly, men are less likely to seek help for depression because it is seen as a weakness, while women are more likely to seek help for the same condition. However, research also shows that for those seen by health professionals, women are more likely to be put on drugs for depression compared to men.[61] In brief, help-seeking behaviour patterns in men and women 'reflect gender-based expectations regarding the perceived differences in vulnerability...'[62]

Treatment Response

Gleaning data from several studies conducted in the West, Pauline M. Prior concludes that 'women more often define problems as "illness" than do men, and health professionals are more likely to medicalize women's problems than men's.'[63] Compared to the West, there appears to be a considerable gap in gendered research from sub-Saharan Africa on mental illness. Notwithstanding that, researchers in Ghana found that 'women are more affected by common mental disorders and are underrepresented in treatment settings'.[64] They concluded on the need for additional research with men or mixed populations to enable them to 'compare the symptoms and correlates of mental distress between men and women'[65] and to be able to scale up mental health services to take care of the large treatment gap. South African researchers, Alison Moultrie and Sharon Kleintjes, also complain that mental health is a generally neglected topic in South Africa. Even more so, women's mental health receives 'little attention in the South African public health sector.'[66] They therefore recommend a wide range of interventions covering psycho-social, cultural and economic empowerment, as well as strengthening women's participation in policy making and other community structures to address women's mental health in South Africa.

Because sex and gender factors are very significant in mental health considerations, some clinicians and researchers insist that these must be taken seriously in both treatment and treatment response. For instance, Burt and Hendrick devote much of the material in their manual to this issue of treatment and response. They underscore the need to pay attention to this process for every identified disorder, working through women's life cycles as well as their vulnerabilities to physical, and socio-biological conditions and events.[67] Some other researchers hold the view that understanding women's mental health, and, indeed, gender differences in mental health requires a framework that goes beyond the narrow medical/scientific model employed primarily by Western researchers to examine the 'dynamics of relationship-driven mental disorders'. This approach recognises that a majority of women most of the time are in relationships with men, and many with their own children or other people's children.[68] They stress the importance of taking into consideration the bio-social and psycho-spiritual aspects of women's mental health issues,[69] particularly within their cultural and locational contexts.

From the foregoing, it is established that serious consideration must be given to the sex and gender dimensions of mental health in diagnosis, treatment and response to treatment. This ensures that both men and women's challenges are examined and attended to in ways that enhance healing and well-being.

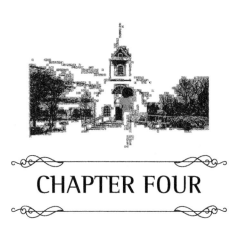

CHAPTER FOUR

HOW CHRISTIAN WOMEN COPE WITH MENTAL HEALTH CHALLENGES AND THE ROLE OF THE CHURCH

Tony Walter astutely observed that 'throughout the modern world, more women than men go to church'.[1] Walter further explains that

> It is, of course, impossible to estimate from behaviour such as going to church or praying daily who might truly be Christian in the eyes of God, but the fact that the more private the devotion, the more likely it is to be a woman who is on her knees, does strongly suggest that female Christians outnumber male Christians even more than female churchgoers outnumber male churchgoers.[2]

The subject of women in the history of Christianity and the Church is not only intriguing and controversial, but also full of paradoxes and ambivalence, especially on the part of the Church. Although women have always been present and active in the life of the Church from its inception in New Testament times, their place, status and role in relation to the Church and Christianity in general have been the subject of much discourse and disagreement, a wide range of differing views and even open conflict among the clergy, laity, the general society and women themselves.[3] These differing views have centred on the interpretation and application of biblical passages on gender relations at home, in church and in society.[4] How these controversies and paradoxes have affected the general health and psychological well-being of women over the centuries, I believe, needs more in-depth investigation by researchers and Christian scholars.

Be that as it may, Christian women like other women also suffer emotional distresses and mental illness, as already established. They are also subject to both the pleasantness and the vicissitudes of life socially, politically, culturally and economically. It appears, however, that being Christian women could be both a factor for positive mental health states and an ability to cope with life's issues. Conversely, it could also serve to undermine their mental health if their Christian self-understanding or the contexts within which they live or operate are deemed unhealthy.[5] By Christian 'self-understanding', I have in mind instances where Christian women themselves interpret biblical texts as a means of self-oppression or subjugation to others. By 'unhealthy contexts', I mean instances (a) where patriarchy operates to bring about domination, violence, discrimination or poverty in ways that negate Christian women's sense of worthiness, well-being, or ability to develop their full capabilities as human beings;[6] (b) where economic and socio-cultural factors also operate to affect the wellbeing of a Christian woman's family, and in turn affect her own mental health; and (c) where Christian religious persons in authority abuse women within that context through manipulation, exploitation, sexual or other forms of abuse, which have grave impacts on their mental wellbeing.

Thus, concerning the issues of self-understanding and unhealthy contexts, Fraser Watts and his colleagues maintain that 'Women use one and half times more medical and psychological resources than men.' And they ask: 'Are women the sicker as well as more religious sex? Or is there something in the way the female role is structured that is unhealthy for women?'[7] Following on the question, they further observe that

> A connection may be made with the 'Christian' virtues that women are socialized to exhibit: submission, dependence, self-effacement, helplessness, emotionality. These patterns can develop into styles of coping that are similar to depressive states... We are forced to conclude that any connection between women's poorer psychological health and Christianity is mediated by a number of factors, especially the prevailing social conditions, and how much support they provide for women...The relationship between Christianity and women's mental health is not simple.[8]

Indeed, as Carol Ann Drogus reports, in the majority world,[9] more women than men appear to seek deeper religious experiences because of their inordinate burdens for the health and upkeep of their children, families and communities. From her observation,

> The broader cultural division of labour into a private, female sphere and a public, male one may also have an impact on women's religious experience. This possibility is glimpsed in descriptions of women as

not only more actively religious but also more emotionally involved and seeking particular kinds of solace from religion.[10]

She affirms that because Latin American women appear to have many more troubles in their concerns for their children, families and relationships, they not only appear to carry more guilt about these issues, but also pray to God more about them. This is an example of how Christian women use their faith as a strong coping mechanism for issues that have implications for their mental wellbeing.

A growing number of studies indicate that African-American women, for example, rely heavily on their religious beliefs and practices to cope with health problems, including depression. Harold K. Koenig reports from one such study of African-American women:

> Religion helped them to integrate negative life events, accept reality, gain insight and courage, confront and transcend limitations, identify and grapple with existential questions, recognize their purpose and destiny, define their character, live their lives within meaningful moral principles, and achieve psychological growth despite difficult circumstances.[11]

This has led to the call to ensure that psychotherapy and other mainstream responses to mental health issues take into serious consideration the role of religion and spirituality, especially in relation to African-Americans whose strong connections to the Christian faith and the historical role of the Black Church in their lives cannot be ignored.[12]

A study on homeless mothers in USA established that 'praying was among the most common strategies used to deal with the difficulties associated with homelessness'.[13] These difficulties included stigma, poverty, stress, anxiety, depression and concerns for their children's welfare. Dana King and others report from another study on Caucasian and African-American middle-aged women that 'attendance at religious services is positively related to subsequent mental health in middle-aged women. The findings support the notion that religious commitment may help mitigate the stress of the midlife period.'[14]

It is interesting to note that in comparison with the Caucasian women in the sample of another study on battered women and the use of spirituality in coping, African-American women were 'significantly more likely to report using prayer as a coping strategy and significantly less likely to seek help from mental health counselors... African-American women found prayer to be more helpful than did the Caucasian women.'[15] Reasons adduced for less use of mental health professionals by the African-American women included their mistrust of the public response system due to the likelihood of racial stigmatisation, the strong emphasis of the private/public dichotomy within the African-American community and the very fact that 'religiosity and spirituality are integral to African-American identity and coping.'[16]

Pastoral leadership obviously has much to do with women's experience of the Church, particularly in their interaction with their local church. Pastors set the agenda, pace and general ethos of church doctrine and practice. If the emotional and mental health issues of a congregation were to be incorporated into pastoral practice, they would relate to the pastor's perception of such issues.

PASTORAL ROLE IN EMOTIONAL AND MENTAL HEALTH RESPONSE

The Christian Church and the clergy have had a long-standing relationship with the issue of care for persons in distress, including mental distress. However, the Church has also been criticised for its turbulent relationship with modern psychology as a discipline, such criticism targeting in particular those of the evangelical tradition. Nevertheless, as pointed out by Howard J. Clinebell, '[M]ental health is a central and inescapable concern of any local church that is a healing-redemptive fellowship.'[17] He thus calls the local church to awake to this mandate:

> In the past, most churches have been like slumbering giants in the area of mental health. If fully awakened, they could release new forces of healing and wholeness in the stream of our world that could turn the tide for the millions of persons toward that fullness of life which is mental health.[18]

Regarding the significant role of pastors or clergy in addressing mental health, Clinebell further asserts:

> The most significant direct contribution of clergymen to mental health is their counseling and shepherding of troubled persons...Troubled people are more apt to seek help from a clergyman than from a member of any other professional group.[19]

The above assertion is actually borne out by a number of studies from different parts of the world on the important role of clergy. In one study of chaplaincy and mental health care in New Zealand, Lindsey B. Carey and Laura del Medico contend that

It can be argued, that clerics and chaplains, through their provision of pastoral care, have been influential in the development of various forms of health care since the time of Constantine...there is evidence that the clergy have been and are still being sought out by those facing personal crisis.[20]

They found in their study that within both 'general mental health and forensic mental health areas, chaplains were often involved in providing spiritual/religious or pastoral assessments about a patient's mental well-being.'[21] They also observed that 'the roles of counselling and education undertaken by chaplaincy personnel seemed substantial and often thematically inseparable from one another.'[22]

Sarah-Louise Hurst's study in the United Kingdom also confirmed the significance of the pastoral role. Regarding her study findings, she states in conclusion:

It has shown how church leaders provide a unique relationship for congregants offering faith, social support and hope... psychology and the Christian faith are very different fields...However, both see themselves as agents of care and healing and share a goal of being compassionate towards those they serve...[23]

Koenig, an expert in faith and mental health issues in the West, also describes the role of clergy and asserts as follows:

Clergy deliver an enormous amount of mental health services to needy persons and families. These mental health services are seldom recognized or acknowledged by mental health professionals, who are often surprised by how much mental health care clergy actually provide. In reality, clergy are often the first line of defense for emotional problems in the population.[24]

It is therefore instructive that Cynthia Franklin and Rowena Fang purposively remind pastors and Church leaders of this role and what they need to be effective:

The people with the greatest needs in our world, such as those in the throes of abuse, poverty, addictions, family crisis, and mental illness, are turning to pastors and church leaders for help. You are empowered by the Holy Spirit to act to heal and deliver, and you can make a decisive difference in a person's recovery and redemption when your actions are guided by both knowledge and compassion.[25]

Franklin and Fang, on their part, succinctly capture this crucial mandate of the Church which had undergirded the call (especially in the West) and underscore the importance, not only for Christian pastors to understand the relationship between religion and mental health, but to also know how this could help them respond in more constructive ways to hurting persons. Mental health practitioners (MHPs) have also begun to understand the need to work with the Church to respond to some of the issues for which patients sought their help. According to Paul B. Maves,

> Ministers increasingly are becoming aware of the relation of religion to mental health and are concerned to discharge more adequately their responsibility for helping persons achieve maturity and maintain mental and emotional equilibrium. At the same time, professional workers in the field of mental health, such as physicians, psychiatrists and psychiatrically oriented social workers are looking increasingly to the Church as an ally in their efforts to help people.[26]

Even though there are currently several views on how much and to what extent the Church and pastors should ignore or integrate psychological knowledge in their response, the calls for such integration have rather intensified.[27] The question, though, remains: what theological background and understanding should be brought to bear on pastoral practice when working with persons affected by emotional and mental distress? In other words, how can the clergy and pastors, including Ghanaian evangelical pastors be helped in exploring the interactions between Christian theology, faith and mental or emotional distress? The subsequent chapters of this book respond to these questions through both the individual experiences of those I interviewed and the theological reflections I bring to bear on the matters examined.

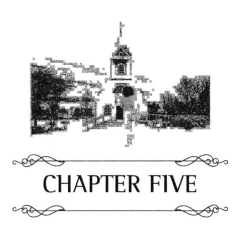

CHAPTER FIVE

OVERVIEW OF MENTAL HEALTH IN GHANA

Ghana's health infrastructure comprises three main sectors: the formal, quasi-formal and informal.[1] The formal consists of government-operated and privately owned hospitals, clinics, health posts, medical laboratories and pharmacies (including church and non-governmental facilities). Three national psychiatric hospitals are included in this sector. The quasi-formal are institutions that provide alternative medical care such as acupuncture, osteopathy and homeopathy clinics and so on. The informal, often termed the traditional medicine sector, includes a diverse array of non-allopathic practitioners, which include herbalists, diviners, soothsayers, bone-setters, as well as healing and miracle-working religious centres or prayer camps.[2]

Ghana's Ministry of Health (MOH) and the Ghana Health Service (GHS) have direct policy supervisory roles over the formal government health sector. The Ministry also has the mandate of forming links with the other sectors to ensure appropriate regulation and the elimination of fake or harmful practices. This role presents a formidable challenge to the MOH and GHS.

A national health insurance scheme is currently in operation and covers attendance at public health and registered private facilities. Although it has made access to health care more accessible and affordable, it is fraught with several operational challenges, including financing.

General Mental Health Data

It is the observation of U.M. Read and V.C.A. Doku that '[P]sychiatry in Ghana is neglected in health care and research.'[3] Although data on the epidemiology of mental disorders in Ghana is 'inadequate and outdated',[4] according to V. de Menil and his co-authors, mental illness represents about 9% of the burden of disease in Ghana.[5] It is estimated that 2.4 to 2.8 million persons in Ghana have mental health challenges, out of which 600,000 have severe mental disabilities.[6]

Public Facilities and Services

Ghana's three national psychiatric hospitals are all based in the southern part of the country.[7] These are the Accra Psychiatric Hospital,[8] the Pantang Hospital and the Ankaful Psychiatric Hospital.[9] However, since 2013, four (4) Regional hospitals have Psychiatric wings which consist of at least 10 to 15 beds, and all district hospitals (required to have 5 virtual beds), now offer mental health services under the Mental Health Decentralization Program which now emphasizes Community Care, a departure from the Institutional Care.[10]

Human Rights Watch reports that private psychiatric hospitals also exist, but 'are too expensive for most Ghanaians.'[11] The School of Medicine and Dentistry of the University of Ghana runs a Department of Psychiatry in Korle-Bu, Accra that also treats persons with mental health challenges. All the public psychiatric hospitals, Human Rights Watch found, are under-staffed, under-funded and do not have enough facilities and logistics to serve the patient population. Although psychiatric medicines are cost-free for patients using the public institutions, there is no social insurance scheme to cover mental disorders. In addition, the hospitals run short of medicines from time to time, causing hardship to patients, caregivers and hospital staff.[12] Community mental health care exists in the country and community psychiatric nurses undergo training for services, but the system is still being developed.[13]

However, it must be recognized that since the establishment of the Mental Health Authority of Ghana and the passage of the Mental Health Act, 2012, mental health data has been improving in terms of numbers of mental health practitioners available to the population, and the government's budgetary allocation for mental health. However the challenges remain ominous in this sector.[14]

Alternative Care and Issues Arising

Writing from the viewpoint of a Western-trained psychiatrist, Margaret Field's study demonstrates how heavily Ghanaians, particularly those in the rural areas, relied on traditional shrines for help with misfortunes, illnesses and mental ill-states in the colonial era, despite the existence of psychiatric hospitals in the country.[15]

Continuing into modern times, many still consult traditional shrines and healing centres, where the methods of spiritual divination (*abisa)* and herbal medicines are combined to treat patients. The concerns raised about traditional treatment include the perceived imprecision of their methods, which could lead to positive or negative results. The Mental Health Act, 2012, attempts to respond to this issue by including traditional practitioners as partners in community care, to ensure they receive basic training and education in mental health issues.

Prayer camps, presumably Christian healing centres, are important players in alternative or complementary care for the emotionally distressed or mentally ill. Some of the camps are set up as 'off-shoots' of some of the spiritual, Pentecostal or Charismatic churches, but often have no direct supervision from their parent churches or from the government.[16] In spite of the apparently increased use of formal health care facilities for the treatment of mental illness than obtained in the past,[17] Olivier Fournier however reported in 2011 that

> [T]he normal pattern for Ghanaians involves utilizing traditional care first and then going to a psychiatric hospital if the problem was not cured. Twenty to thirty percent of the Accra Psychiatric Hospital's patients try spiritual or traditional healing before a family member or the court brings them to the psychiatric hospital. About 20% of patients use faith healing after leaving the hospital for spiritual reinforcement.[18]

Obviously, more research is needed to confirm or disprove these trends and assertions. If such 'spiritual reinforcement' is sought also from evangelical Ghanaian pastors, then it makes the underlying assumption of this study even more significant; that is, what will be the nature of the help that these pastors give to those who seek them for such?

Socio-cultural Issues, Stigma and Social Responses

In Ghana, 'evil spirits and demons'[19] are widely considered, even by those who are affected, to cause mental illness. Adages and proverbs depicting the social perceptions of mental challenges and the stigma of mental illness exist in Ghanaian languages. In Ga language, for example, sɛkɛ means 'madness' or 'insanity'. Anyone who is seen misbehaving or going contrary to socially accepted norms is asked, *'Oye sɛkɛ alo?'*, meaning, 'Are you going mad?' In the Twi (Akan) language, *abɔdam* refers to the state of a person who is mentally ill. Again, people who misbehave, whether mentally ill or not, are asked, *'Wa bɔ dam?'* meaning, 'Are you mad?' This shows the equation of mental illness with social unacceptability. The Akan believe that families with mentally challenged people are not eligible for marriage and respectable families do not marry from them.[20] Families generally consider their mentally ill relatives to be a disgrace to them.[21] Someone who has recovered from mental illness is still viewed with suspicion and the Akan comment is '*Kakra a yɛ de hunahuna nkwadaa deɛ ebi da so wɔ mu*' (literally, 'Even if the person has recovered, there is still a bit of illness remaining that can be used to scare children.').

Nurses and doctors who work at public mental health facilities are also stigmatised as having contracted by association the disease of their patients.[22] Many families abandon their mentally challenged relatives in the psychiatric hospitals and prayer camps, considering their care too much of a burden and fearing the societal stigma on the family.[23] Often, patients who have received treatment at the psychiatric hospitals are afraid to go back to their communities because of the stigma and rejection.[24]

Human Rights Watch also documented 'severe cases of physical and verbal abuse of persons with mental disabilities in the family, community, and hospitals and prayer camps.'[25] Ghanaian children with mental disabilities do not fare any better than adults. Whether afflicted with neurologically based illnesses such as Down's syndrome, or autism, epilepsy or other mental illness, they and their families are stigmatised.[26] In some parts of northern Ghana, children born with severe disabilities including mental illness are believed to be 'spirit-children',[27] and are put to death or abandoned and left to die.

Policy and Legislative Issues

A few months after passing a new Mental Health Act, 2012 (Act 846),[28] Ghana ratified the UN Convention on the Rights of Persons with Disability[29] in July 2012. Before the Act, the legislation that existed, titled Mental Health Decree, 1972,[30] was totally inadequate in dealing with the myriad issues that needed to be addressed. In fact, the Decree was not implemented for forty years.[31] The 2012 Act attempts to address many of the issues identified as necessary for treatment, such as stigma, discrimination and abuse, while decentralising care and treatment largely through community response. It established a Mental Health Authority (MHA) with the mandate to coordinate all mental health issues. It also set up an independent Mental Health Fund for providing financial resources for the care and management of persons with mental illness.[32] Other provisions include the establishment of a Mental Health Review Tribunal to deal among other things with involuntary admissions and long-term voluntary admissions, employment rights, protection of vulnerable groups such as women, children and the aged, guardianship and psycho-social rehabilitation.

Ghana's general lacklustre performance in the implementation of socially-related legislation however makes continuous advocacy, monitoring and evaluation imperative to ensure that the law does not suffer inadequate attention and implementation. This is especially important because even though Ghana's mental health policy was in place since 2007, a lack of resources prevented many of the goals from being reached.[33] However, the Mental Health Authority has developed and adopted a ten-year plan for Ghana (2018-2027). It is hoped that this plan would receive adequate budgetary support for its full implementation.[34]

ADVOCACY AND MOBILISATION FOR PROMOTING MENTAL HEALTH ISSUES

Ghana does have consumer associations for people with mental disorders. Generally speaking, Government agencies, NGOs, professional associations and International agencies have promoted public education and awareness campaigns. However, with the passage of the Act, the Mental Health Authority is now mandated to coordinate education and awareness campaigns. Also in existence is the Mental Health Society of Ghana (MEHSOG), a countrywide association of persons with mental disorders and epilepsy who use mental health services. Formed in 2009, it aims to fight for the rights of the mentally challenged to influence policy making for their appropriate treatment and care.[35] An NGO that has led several advocacy efforts, including that for the passage of the Mental Health Act and coordinated MESHOG's formation and work is BasicNeeds, Ghana. BasicNeeds' programme initiatives also integrate economic livelihood empowerment for the users.[36]

As alluded to above, several weaknesses have been identified in the system that needs to be addressed. These include
- Very low budgeting for mental health
- Over-centralisation of formal services
- Neglect in implementation of legislation, policies and plans
- Inadequate planning, monitoring, service and quality improvement
- Widespread breach of human rights in mental health care facilities, whether formal or traditional/faith-based facilities
- Inconsistent supply and shortages of medication in facilities
- Inadequate supervision and monitoring of faith-based and traditional healing practitioners and centres
- Inadequate training in human rights for mental healthcare providers across board
- Treatment too strongly focused on medication rather than other psycho-social interventions

- Free treatment is a myth and there is no insurance cover for medication
- Not enough attention and logistics for children with mental challenges
- Insufficient public education
- Very few doctors willing to train in mental health
- Policy-makers do not take mental health seriously enough
- Inadequate research and disaggregated data[37]

Many of these weaknesses are also outlined in the Human Rights Watch Report *'Like a Death Sentence'*, even though they are analysed from a human rights framework perspective, with emphasis on abuses within the existing formal and informal systems.[38]

Much effort has gone into making critical recommendations for improving the system of mental healthcare in Ghana and the elimination of abuse and discrimination. These include the need to implement the 2012 Act and its related policies and plans, strengthen the collaboration between the formal mental health system and the work of churches, faith-based and traditional healing practitioners, as well as the need to harmonise and integrate their practices with the standards outlined in the Mental Health Act.[39]

SOME WOMEN'S HEALTH ISSUES THAT IMPINGE ON WOMEN'S MENTAL HEALTH IN GHANA

Maternal Mortality

Women's health in Ghana is a serious national concern. Both men and women have a wide range of health issues stemming from communicable and non-communicable diseases, but maternity and reproductive health matters compound women's challenges. Although the government has developed some strategies to address these, maternal mortality, for example, remains unacceptably high, with an average of 319 deaths in 100,000 live births, even though this is seen as a drop from much higher figures in past years.[40]

Ghana's National Gender Policy states that 'A large number of women are dying annually because of pregnancy related complications, severe bleeding...hypertensive diseases, infections and unsafe abortions.'[41] Fertility is relatively high and the use of contraception quite low. The GSS reports that 'Nearly four out of every five women aged 15-49 years or their partners were not using any form of contraceptive method.'[42] HIV/AIDS among women, which has grave implications for mental wellbeing, also remains a challenge, although overall prevalence rates in the country have been significantly reduced.[43] The emotional and psychological toll of all of these health challenges on the affected Ghanaian women cannot be ignored.

Violence against Women in Ghana

The state of violence against women and girls in Ghana is captured starkly in the situational analysis section of Ghana's *National Gender Policy*. It states that

> Violence against women and human trafficking is a major...problem in Ghana that needs more aggressive and a quicker policy response. The high incidents of rape and other sexual offences from the (Domestic Violence and Victim Support Unit) DOVVSU records is alarming. There is the need for ...action to curb the prevalence of rape, sexual abuse, serial women and wives killings, maiming and human trafficking.[44]

In a Ghanaian study, Adomako Ampofo and her co-researchers comment specifically on the issue of marital violence and how society employs culture to silence women:

> The abuse of spouses is all about power and control. Cultural wisdom such as: "marriage is a long journey"; "for a marriage to succeed, one partner should be [a] fool"; "a woman should 'hold her nose' and stay in the marriage for the sake of the children", is expressed in every Ghanaian language especially as 'guidelines' to all women: from the young unmarried to the married...These 'guidelines' to a successful marriage are expected to be adhered to...only the unwise woman disregards them. The reporting of violence by female spouses to the police then becomes 'uncalled for' and should be done only as a last resort.[45]

The study found that in Ghana, there are many reasons why the perpetrators of violence against women escape formal prosecution. These include the general poverty status of victims, lack of information regarding institutions that can help, obstructions in the legal processes, including bias of officials, uncooperative attitude of witnesses in the community, as well as collusion between the victims, victims' families and perpetrators to drop the cases, among others.[46] These reasons still exist despite legal provisions in both the Criminal and Other Offences Act[47] and the Domestic Violence Act[48] to address such violence.[49] The costs and inimical effects of violence on women's health and mental health cannot be underrated. For example, sexual violence increases women's risks of contracting HIV/AIDS and other sexually transmitted infections. HIV/AIDS also exposes women to greater societal stigma and dispossession of subsistence or property.[50] These factors in turn make women more vulnerable to mental ill-health.

Women's Disability Status

According to the Ghana Statistical Service (GSS), women with disability are more 'likely to experience public spaces as intimidating and dangerous'[51] and are also likely to be poorer than men with disability.[52] Women with disability face serious discrimination, especially when it comes to marriage, and are also often impregnated by unscrupulous males and left to fend for themselves and their children.[53] Without doubt therefore, women with mental disabilities face all these restrictions, stigma and more in Ghana.

WOMEN'S MENTAL HEALTH IN GHANA

Ghana has several laws, policies and institutions dedicated to the promotion of women's rights, empowerment and wellbeing. However, practical implementation of such laws and operationalisation of policies are still inadequate. Socio-cultural attitudes regarding women's personhood and status still somewhat challenge women's empowerment, regardless of the gains made in women's educational, social and economic status.[54] Nonetheless, a full discussion of women's rights and empowerment is beyond the remit of this study. Suffice it to say that the socio-cultural, legal, political and economic contexts have various ramifications for Ghanaian women's health, mental health and emotional wellbeing. Where women's needs and rights are recognised and upheld in family, church/religious spaces and society, there are, generally, positive implications for women's mental wellbeing. The reverse in any of these spheres of endeavour is likely to result in a negative impact on women's emotional and mental health.

A review of the relevant literature shows that not much research has been done on women and their mental health needs in Ghana. Yet, the few studies that currently exist contain significant data to present a fair understanding of women's mental health issues in the country. A significant number of women face mental distress and illness in Ghana. Heather Sipsma and her colleagues concluded from their Ghanaian study conducted among a large, nationally representative sample, that the prevalence of psychological distress was higher among women than men.[55]

Thus while Ghanaian women suffer from all the diagnostic categories of mental disorders, it appears women form the majority of patients with depression in Ghana   Margaret Field's 1930s study in the Akan rural areas of Ghana mentions that '[D]epression is the commonest mental illness of Akan rural women....'[56] However women are also sufferers of schizophrenia, schizotypal and delusional disorders, anxiety and other forms of mental distress and illness.

Notwithstanding that, the fact that women suffer depression in significant proportions is consistent with what Dr Akwasi Owusu Osei, former Chief Psychiatrist of Ghana and currently the Chief Executive Officer of the Mental Health Authority in Ghana, said in my interview with him. As Chief Psychiatrist, he claimed to have treated slightly more females than males, with depression largely characterising the symptoms for females.[57] Dr Ama Edwin, Medical Practitioner and a Clinical Psychologist, then at the Korle-Bu Hospital, Accra also reported treating more females than males, with the former reporting more depression and anxiety-related symptoms.[58] There is therefore the need for more exploratory studies into Ghanaian women's particular disposition towards depression to determine whether, like other studies elsewhere, there is a multiplicity of contributory factors, or whether there are particularly notable issues within the Ghanaian context that pre-dispose women to depression.

With respect to women's access to care, Read and Doku report that

Women in Ghana appear to be underserved by mental health services, and the majority of women suffering from mental disorders, particularly depression, remain untreated or under the care of churches and shrines. Research at facilities such as polyclinics, shrines and churches may provide a more accurate picture of the numbers of women with mental disorders and their clinical representation.[59]

Perceptions about Ghanaian Women with Mental and Emotional Distress

Angela Ofori-Atta and her co-researchers conducted an important study into the common understandings and perceptions of Ghanaians about Ghanaian women with mental problems.[60] In brief, they found that all the respondents believed that more women than men were affected by mental illness, particularly depression.[61] Also, they gave divergent explanations regarding the possible causes of women's mental illness, including women being the weaker sex, hormonal problems, unfulfilled emotional expectations of love from men, adultery, witchcraft, physical abuse, infertility and poverty. These supposed causes were clustered under three broad categories as inherent vulnerability, witchcraft and gender disadvantage.[62]

Several respondents in the Ofori-Atta study (including general health and mental health practitioners) believed women to be naturally and essentially pre-disposed to mental illness. They used phrases such as 'weaker', 'less self-reliant', 'dependent on men', 'unable to cope with frustrations' and so on to buttress their claims.[63] They also believed that women 'naturally anticipate too much from marriage and relationships',[64] leading to their disappointment and distress. Respondents within the health sector stressed the fundamental role that hormonal changes play in women's mental health issues.[65]

The respondents in the Ofori-Atta-led study also recognised that gendered forms of social disadvantage affect women's mental health and wellbeing. They mentioned polygamy and extra-marital affairs by husbands, physical abuse and poverty as significant concerns that also endanger their health in the country.[66] The silence on domestic and other forms of abuse of women were also of concern to respondents in the study, especially considering how such abuse could trigger mental ill-health symptoms in women.[67] Abuse also featured significantly in the Sipsma-led study, which found that women who reported physical abuse, increased partner control and were acceptable to women's disempowerment had a greater likelihood of psychological distress.[68]

Poverty also emerged as a significant factor in Ghanaian women's mental distress states. Women who are denied autonomy and agency in financial affairs in their families, or are dependent on men for their source of finances are also affected in their mental health.[69] One worrisome finding was the linkage between poverty and young women's mental health, due to possible economic exploitation from older men.[70]

Ofori-Atta and her co-authors concluded from their survey that there is the need to recognise that 'improving women's mental health in Ghana and other low-income countries may require intersectoral work and policies that prioritize gender mainstreaming in order to improve the economic, cultural and social status of women.'[71] To corroborate this point, de Menil, Osei and others emphatically affirm that '...certain social factors – in particular, education, employment and income – play an important role in the mental health of urban Ghanaian women. These social factors should be taken into consideration in both the prevention and treatment of mental disorders.'[72]

A Note on Depression (and other Mental Disorders) in Ghanaian Women and the Connection with Witchcraft

The study by Ofori-Atta and her co-researchers also revealed that the respondents believe that the Ghanaian community views mental illness in both women and men as the work of witches these witches being mainly women themselves. It highlighted that very often, women suspected of using witchcraft to 'cause mental problems are expelled from the community, particularly in northern Ghana...'[73] These women are 'forced to move to designated places, or "witchcamps".[74] As the researchers aptly state from their findings, 'Women are frequently blamed for the mental illness in the community, and are consequently "pathologized" and relegated to a life of rejection and isolation.'[75]

There have been cases in Ghana where some women experience the perception or accusation of being witches. There are also situations where women go through emotional or mental distress and as a result, perceive themselves as witches. In the latter case, for example, Margaret Field found in the cases she documented from the Mframaso shrine in the Ashanti Region that nearly all the female patients with depression came to the shrines with spontaneous self-accusations of witchcraft, that is, of having caused harm without a concrete act or conscious will.[76] Field also observed the social standing and achievements of the women reporting symptoms of depression as follows:

> In rural Ghana, Involutional Depression with agitation is ... one of the commonest and most clearly defined of mental illnesses. The majority of patients are conscientious women of good personality who have worked hard and launched a fleet of well-brought-up children. Many of them have paid for their children's schooling with money earned by diligent trading, gardening or cocoa-farming.[77]

Making the connections between women's mental distress and their status in marriage, particularly during their menopausal stages, Field continued:

> In Ghana, the patient has the additional stress of seeing her husband take on [an] extra and younger wife so that he may continue to beget children... Most women, quite apart from depressives, are worried by these social hazards of the menopause, and many of them, when they become aware of amenorrhea, go from shrine to shrine over several years with the plaint (sic) 'I am pregnant but the pregnancy doesn't grow.'[78]

Thus, the distress states caused by hormonal and social status changes increase women's vulnerability to self-accusation and witch accusation from the community because of the pervasive belief in the supernatural causes of illness or distress symptoms.

In Ghana, therefore, it appears the phenomenon of witchcraft and its association with women's mental illness plays out in a number of ways: (a) a woman voluntarily (or involuntarily) confesses to being a witch, possibly because of her mental health status; (b) a woman is accused of being a witch leading to her becoming mentally disturbed; and (c) a woman accuses another woman of being a witch, and, in this case, the accuser herself may be having mental health challenges which may have led to the accusation in the first place.

Some MHPs and community advocates, though, attempt to explain these possible scenarios, all of which have mental health implications. An ACTIONAID Report states, for instance, that

> Witchcraft accusations also stem from a lack of recognition or treatment for mental health issues. According to Dr Akwesi (sic) Osei, chief psychiatrist in the Ghana Health Service… women who are accused of witchcraft are often suffering from clinical depression, schizophrenia or dementia[79]

Dr Akwasi Osei has also researched the link between witchcraft and depression, and examines the incidence of depression among 17 self-confessed witches at three shrines in the Ashanti Region of Ghana. Using the WHO ICD-10 standards, he found that they were all depressed. Three of the women also had serious physical illnesses. In his study, the self-confessed witches complained of 'burning sensations' and persistent headaches, as well as expressing guilt at having used witchcraft to harm people in their families. Osei's findings from this study are similar to those found in Margaret Field's work, namely, that the inexplicable experiences and feelings of guilt that women especially go through when ill with depression lead to confessions of witchcraft.[80] Thus, whether self-confessed or accused by others, it is essential to factor mental health implications into situations where women specifically face this phenomenon.

In his study on Akan witchcraft, Opoku Onyinah postulates that although Western psychological and social instability theories could account for self-accusation or other-accusation of witchcraft, it is vital not to discount the Akan traditional concept of *Abisa*the strong and pervasive belief in the causality of misfortune and ill-health, as well as people's pursued search for stability in one's destiny. This belief leads many, whether believers in African traditional religion or Christians, to interpret illness in the community or one's own ill-health as the work of evil forces such as witchcraft. This, in turn, leads to the desperate search for an antidote from traditional anti-witchcraft shrines or the Christian prayer camps.[81] Further research and public sensitisation on the various scenarios are needed because of the serious impact on women's lives and the deep divisions and disruptions such accusations generate in families and communities. Without doubt, the status of mental health and women's mental health in Ghana raises significant questions for researchers, practitioners and even women themselves. Ensuring that women, in particular, have sound mental health has far reaching ramifications for the health not only of families, but also even of communities. I now turn to the Ghanaian Christian women who experienced various degrees of emotional/mental distress or illnesses, to present what they had to say about their experiences and the kind of help they received from different sources; in particular, the help from their own pastors and other pastors they consulted in their bid to find a solution.

CHAPTER SIX

GHANAIAN CHRISTIAN WOMEN'S EXPERIENCES OF MENTAL HEALTH CHALLENGES AND THEIR PERSPECTIVES ON RESPONSES

Introduction

I interviewed Ten (10) Christian women survivors for this study.[1] Their selection was based on the following criteria: (a) they were adult women[2]; (b) they were all evangelical Christians; (c) they had survived or were still experiencing emotional or mental distress or illness; and (d) they could articulate their experiences and views well. I wanted to explore their thoughts, emotions, perceptions, views, beliefs and attempts to make meaning of their peculiar mental health challenges.

Although these women hailed from different parts of the country and belonged to different ethnic groups, they were all resident in Accra, the capital of Ghana. Their average age was 47 years, with the youngest at 32 years and the eldest aged 62. Three of the respondents were members of the Church of Pentecost (COP), two were from Lighthouse Chapel International (LCI), two were Anglican, one Presbyterian, one Methodist and the last considered herself a Charismatic Christian. Their educational backgrounds ranged from below the first degree (Junior High School, Certificate and Diploma holders), to the first degree (in a university or equivalent institution) and postgraduate degrees (Master's degree and above). The lowest level of education was Junior High School certificate (10%), and the highest percentage comprised degree holders (40%), followed by postgraduate/Master's degree level (30%), and Teacher Training Certificate 'A' (20%). Two out of the ten were married, three were single/never married, one was widowed, one separated and two divorced. Some respondents had lived with their mental illness/emotional distress for the past 35 years, being the longest period recorded in the study. The shortest period of illness however was 9 years. For the purposes of anonymity, each respondent was assigned a number (1, 2, 3, etc.) in the order in which they were interviewed. I also assigned each a pseudo name for confidentiality purposes.

Table 9: Profile of Christian Women Survivors Interviewed

Respondent	Age	Marital Status	Educational level	Period of distress	Formal Diagnosis
1 (Amma)	36	Single	Graduate	From 1995	Bipolar
2 (Akua)	59	Widowed	Graduate	From 1978	Bipolar
3 (Naki))	51	Married	Postgraduate	From 1989	Obsessive Compulsive Disorder (OCD)
4 (Adjo)	49	Separated	Postgraduate	From 2000	Depression
5 (Bema)	45	Married	Below first degree	2007 - 2011	Not told
6 (Korkor)	32	Single	Below first degree	From about 1994	Obsessive Compulsive Disorder (OCD)
7 (Serwa)	52	Divorced	Postgraduate	From 2000	Depression
8 (Rita)	62	Widowed	Below first degree	From 1982	Schizophre-nia
9 (Efua)	45	Divorced	Below first degree	From 2007	Not told
10 (Kaaley)	32	Single	Below first degree	2001-2005	Depression

All the interviews were conducted in English, with the exception of one where the respondent gave answers in both English and Twi.

Nine (9) major themes emerged from the women's responses. These themes are broken down as follows: i) perceptions of causes of their emotional/ mental ill-health; ii) description of symptoms; iii) perception of connection between condition and femaleness; iv) societal attitudes and responses to their condition; and v) help-seeking; and specific pastoral responses from evangelical Ghanaian pastors (EGPs). The other themes are vi) personal faith and spirituality as coping mechanisms; vii) collaboration between pastoral response and mental health professionals (MHPs); and viii) perspectives and recommendations for improvement in pastoral response.

Perceptions of Causes of Respondents' Emotional/Mental Ill-health

The ten women interviewed identified a range of the possible causes of their conditions. Some were immediate and others more remote. Primary among the causes for the women was the spiritual factor. That notwithstanding, they also pointed to other causes encompassing social, medical, childhood and other factors.

a. *Spiritual causality/connection*
It was not surprising that eight (80%) of the women sufferers/respondents, being African and Ghanaian, believed that there was a link between mental illnesses/emotional distresses and spiritual factors or forces, as Akua, (Respondent 2) put it, '... for me, every sickness has a spiritual part...' Reinforcing this view, Kaaley (Respondent 10) believed also that malevolent forces operating from her family background caused her condition:

> As a Christian, I believe that for anything to happen physically, it has to occur in the spiritual realm before it occurs... From what people, the men and women of God were saying, that something that [is] coming from the back of my mother and father's families... *(Kaaley)*

For Rita, who was Respondent 8, it was the nature of the experience and the accompanying frightening symptoms that convinced her of the spiritual linkage:

> Somebody will have something like hallucination, hearing voices, seeing things that we cannot comprehend; it's the spiritual one and you cannot do anything...

Korkor, (Respondent 6) explained her condition by searching for meaning in biblical texts that describe Christians wrestling with forces of darkness:

> Our wrestling is not with flesh and blood, but with principalities and authorities. So at times, the devil may get chance to do this...

Also, self-blame and guilt for sins committed in the past haunted Naki, Respondent 3 who expressed her distress in spiritual terms:

> I thought something was happening to me spiritually and so I attributed it to the particular past sin that I committed for which this is my punishment.

Two respondents, Amma and Efua, however believed the contrary about the element of spiritual causality or connection:

> In my personal opinion, mental illness and spiritual, like demons, they can be related but I think they are two different things... *(Amma)*

> You know maybe those that may have offended the deities, but most of it is sickness and physical things that happen to people that disturbs them mentally...*(Efua)*

The women were also quite clear about the other factors they perceived to have caused or precipitated their conditions. These range from various forms of social stressors, childhood abuse, marital and family issues and medical factors. In some cases, they cited a multiplicity of causes. Six (60%) of them clearly identified dysfunctional marriage/romantic relationships as having caused or aggravated their condition. The following extracts throw more light on these other factors:

b. *Stress*
Two respondents specifically referred to stressful situations triggering off their mental challenges:

> It happens when I'm under a very stressful situation...The first time I was preparing for my A-Level examinations which was quite stressful. So I think that was what triggered it. The subsequent episodes that I have had, I always have myself getting a relapse when am in a very stressful environment...*(Amma)*

Adjo, (Respondent 4) appeared to have multiple stressors acting together to add to her misery during her experience. In her case, Adjo believed the care obligations of her nuclear and extended family aggravated her condition:

> I felt obliged to take care of my sister's children because their mother isn't here, their father died and all those other things from family. Pressures here and there, my brother living with me for eleven years because he had had a stroke...

Susan Kornstein and Barbara Wojcik confirm that women are more likely than men to experience the onset of depression when stressful life events occur, as they respond to stressors from their family, children and reproductive difficulties.[3] Angela B. McBride also points out how managing multiple roles between professional, family and community responsibilities place a strain on women.[4] This certainly was the case with Adjo, when her professional ambitions stalled:

> ...[n]ot completing my PhD for my career progression was also haunting me. So I started having panic attacks upon panic attacks until this day.

I was not surprised therefore when during our interview, Adjo burst into tears with the plea, 'I wish I had someone to help me. I have taken care of everybody but myself.'

c.   *Marital and Relationship problems*

The perception that women place a premium on their relationships with men was manifestly evident in this study.[5] Five of the six respondents who attributed their experience to failed romantic/marital relationships narrated how they happened. For Korkor, the sixth respondent, difficulties in her marriage worsened her condition due to the neglect she faced from her husband, although she attributed her mental illness to another factor. Below are excerpts from the five women on the perceived triggers or contributors to their mental illness. Three of them experienced heartbreaks from failed relationships:

> I felt at that age...why a man would say he didn't want to marry me, and so I thought about it and it brought about an episode... the broken heart triggered it. *(Amma)*

> ...[b]reaking up with my boyfriend of six years because we didn't agree on the abortion. He wanted me to keep the pregnancy and my father didn't want me to keep the pregnancy...*(Akua)*

> I had a broken relationship with my children's father and for me, marriage was something I really lived for and I was not ready for a life as a single mother... I started feeling lonely. *(Adjo)*

For Respondent 7, Serwa, the trigger was her husband's infidelity:
> My husband then was studying in a ... (foreign country) and those white girls; he was following them.

Rita, on the other hand, pointed to unrequited love or the perception of being jilted by a potential suitor:

> I was praying for a husband. By then (name withheld) he was a young priest then so we were friends. I thought we were going to get married but...

d.   *Childhood neglect or abuse*

These responses illustrate Husna Razee's findings, namely, that women recognise the paradoxes in their relationships with men.[6] On the one hand, men provided security, social respect, financial support and companionship in marriage, while on the other, they were the cause of much heartache and emotional unhappiness within or outside marriage.

Three (30%) of the respondents related incidents of childhood abuse or neglect, which they linked to the development of mental illness during childhood or later in life. The possibility is very real that being exposed to such conditions could have been the contributory factor to their experience:

> I was staying with my aunty who used metal bucket on my head so that created that problem that worried me for years. *(Efua)*

> I was not treated well among my siblings. There was no love. So I am that type that nobody understands so they started ignoring me... *(Rita)*

> He (my father) beat us without reason. We have no right to play with other children as other children play...he inflicted fear in us that we can't go out when he is around and we don't feel free... *(Kaaley)*

Bruce L. Levin and Marian A. Becker have suggested a strong causal relationship between poor mental health and childhood events involving psychological, physical or sexual abuse.[7] It is disheartening that apart from the physical abuse she faced from her father, Kaaley had also suffered sexual abuse during her childhood. She summarised her ordeal in a terse statement on which she would not elaborate during the interview:

> ...[t]hree times raped and all by trusted family friends...

e.   *Medical/biological /genetic causes*

The women's responses lend credence to the possibility of multiple causes of the onset of mental illnesses. Three of the respondents, who mentioned social stressors or spiritual connections, also believed that genetic and biological factors could have accounted for their condition:

Maybe I was that already because I remember when I was in school, sometimes I used to get the report that I was erratic...*(Akua)*

I had a total abdominal hysterectomy which took away my body's ability to produce estrogen naturally and it actually changed my hormonal system. It started making me feel very miserable...*(Adjo)*

But I think my mother also... She also suffered mental illness; she was also admitted at the Accra psychiatric hospital....*(Kaaley)*

Taken together with other responses, these answers require that help-givers such as medical and mental health practitioners, as well as pastoral caregivers and counsellors, have to be cautious about drawing quick and over-simplistic conclusions about causality, because of the complex pathways of mental illness.[8] It remains to be seen how this caution could influence the kind of response and help given to persons with mental illness.

Manifesting Symptoms

Three out of the ten respondents were diagnosed with clinical depression, two with bipolar disorder, two with Obsessive Compulsive Disorder (OCD), one with schizophrenia and two were not told their diagnoses. Even those who were not sure of their diagnoses were able to clearly describe the symptoms of their conditions, as their responses indicate below. For example, the two OCD survivors, described theirs in part as follows:

I couldn't tell them that I was insulting God in my head and those things...*(Naki)*

When I am going to bathe, I have to scrub myself repetitively. I have to wash myself in patterns and all that keeps long. The way I bath, I have to be going up and down for a long time. And when I am washing too, the same thing. When I finish washing, a thought comes into my mind that it is not well done. Or you did not even do it at all, then I am compelled and forced to wash it again...*(Korkor)*

One of the clinical depression survivors described her symptoms thus:

I couldn't sleep and for about three days, I did not sleep and I kept visiting the health post but every time I went the doctor was not there... I was depressed I think and then I could not do certain things again like cooking, washing, and reading. ... I felt dull, I always want to be alone and shy away from people...*(Kaaley)*

Amma aptly described the cyclical nature of bipolar disorder and the way it distorts behaviour and perception:

> In the hyper state, you want to go out, spend a lot of money, you want to make friends, you always want to see the world, and I can talk on the phone for hours to everybody... In the depressive state, you become complete opposite, all you want to do is sleep, you are lethargic...

Even though three of them were formally diagnosed with depression, other co-morbid conditions could have been present, for it is known that depression often accompanies other illnesses, for example, bipolar disorder (which actually has a depressive side) and OCD.[9] A depressed mind may lead to suicidal thoughts, which a significant number of the respondents had, with a few making actual attempts:

> I did try to commit suicide in the year 2000. I just felt so down and so out, so worthless, so useless...*(Amma)*

> Sometimes I would have to admit to being suicidal so many times ... emotionally, am not strong anymore. *(Adjo)*

For Naki, threatening to actually commit the act of suicide brought about a much needed intervention from a hospital at the time:
> [W]hen I went there and I said I wanted to kill myself, he made me see Dr Asare.

Akua found a remarkable way of coping with suicidal ideation:
> When I have suicide thoughts, I talk to God.

That many mentally ill persons, including Christians, have suicidal ideation and some even attempt suicide requires both deep theological reflection as well as sensitive and informed pastoral response and care. It was beyond the scope of this study to examine the psychology of suicide, or to do a theological appraisal of the phenomenon. The response, however, is not stern rebuke, criminalisation of failed attempts or shaming the mentally ill sufferer, but rather attentive, loving care from family, loved ones and sensitive caregivers, including pastors. One can only begin to understand the kind of despair that these women were facing. Writing about her own pain of depression, author Sheila Walsh describes her challenge: 'I wanted so much to be able to pull myself together, but how do you hold a mountain in place when it is crumbling from inside?'[10] One also hears the cries of these women through Kathryn Greene-McCreight's own words to God in her deep despair: '[R]ebuke the winds, calm the waves, still the chaos within...you who at creation calmed the stormy waters by creating the land... dear Word of God, in me create islands of peace, foothills in the midst of the raging sea.'[11]

Perceived Connection between Mental Illness and Femaleness

In answering the question, 'In your opinion, did your mental illness have anything to do with your being a woman?', five respondents did not find any connection between their mental illness and their femaleness. Here are two of the reasons given:

> I don't think so, it's more of my frame, like my whole body constitution, I am one who is prone to mood swings...*(Naki)*

> As for me, all my life, like when I was in sixth form, we were only two girls in a class of men so I have never had that feeling that any thing is happening to me because I am a woman...*(Akua)*

The other three who answered 'Yes' to this question also gave their reasons for thinking that their femaleness was connected to the mental illness they suffered. Amma and Adjo explained it in terms of biology combined with gender expectations, as seen in the extracts of their responses below:

> My first episode that happened when I was seventeen and I was told at that time it was a puberty thing. Since I was entering puberty, it was a hormonal sickness and those of us who may have pains at seventeen to eighteen, it happens because of you being a woman...*(Amma)*

> [I]t's because I'm a woman that I feel the need for a man's love and the woman in me has always sought that...So it makes me vulnerable. I also feel that being a mother, which is also part of being a woman, makes me equally vulnerable because I don't know how to neglect the people in my care. I am the last person to think of myself. It's what women do. *(Adjo)*

Mental health and illness interact with both sex and gender factors. Both factors are a consistent thread the runs through the women's experiences, even for those who believed the onset of their condition had nothing to do with their sex. They still had to deal with gendered attitudes and stereotypes in both the places where they sought help and in society. This was the experience of Respondent 2, Akua, who was accused of being a witch at a *sunsum sɔre*:[12]

[T]his man too, because I challenged him, he said I was a witch. So one Sunday, my father came to church and they made me strip and I was left with only my panty in front of the whole church...

Societal Attitudes and Responses to their Condition of Mental Illness

The respondents experienced various attitudes from their families and members of the society. On the one hand, there was sympathy and support, primarily from some family members and caregivers. Three of the women stated:

So when an uncle of mine heard that this was the situation, he volunteered to buy my medication for me all the time. *(Amma)*

But... (my friend) also opened my eyes that there are solutions that this problem can be dealt with. *(Korkor)*

When I was admitted in Kumasi, my elder sister took care of me there and the other siblings also... He (husband) came there all the way from Salaga to Kumasi and back at least every week...praying all the time. *(Bema)*

On the other hand, most of them experienced painful stigma, scorn, fear and sometimes discrimination or exclusion, as illustrated in the four responses below:

When you become well and you feel you can contribute effectively to family issues, they feel that you have this problem so when we are talking about certain things you shouldn't come in. *(Amma)*

When I finished (eating), they threw the bowl away. Immediately I knew that I was not considered normal. I realized that people do not want to associate with me... that one was really painful to me. *(Akua)*

A senior pastor in the ...church was the one who preached during the wedding. And he said a woman without a husband has no honour in our society. In fact, it hit me; even worse, it pierced my heart... *(Adjo)*

I saw the Sunday school teachers didn't want me to get close to them... When that happens, it hurts me very much... *(Rita)*

The women largely internalised the negative experiences of guilt, shame, isolation, fear and sometimes felt abandoned by God. They also went through self-stigmatisation. All of these emotions were symptomatic of the distress they were suffering:

> I lost me, and not recovering me has been the major challenge in my life. I miss me. *(Adjo)*

> [T]he way my mother has suffered, I want to make her happy and be proud. I am not able to achieve it. And am not able to let the younger ones also look up to me and better their lives...*(Korkor)*

> I had concluded that I was going to hell because of the thing that was happening to me. I mean, how can I have another person's name on my lips and in my mind when Jesus is supposed to be Lord of my heart? Certainly, either I have witchcraft or something. *(Naki)*

> So I will be indoors for some time and all that I was doing was praying. I was always praying, reading my Bible. Lord, forgive me if I have sinned in any way. *(Bema)*

Kaaley, who said that three family friends sexually assaulted her in her childhood, had developed a deep-seated anger, which she acted out later in life:

> I felt broken. So from then I started using the mindset of a tomboy because now I needed to fight men. I think all other men are same and have done same thing to women...

The account by Naki above echoes the mental confusion created by distress and which leads women to sometimes accuse themselves of witchcraft. In fact, the feelings Kaaley also expressed are not unusual. Vivien K. Burt and Victoria C. Hendrick explain that over a longer term, women who have experienced sexual assault feel 'out of control, ashamed, vulnerable, guilty and depressed.'[13] They maintain that these often experience 'sexual dysfunction and aversion and may have difficulty maintaining healthy interpersonal relationships.'[14]

Seeking Help

From the perspective of Christian women, the themes of seeking help and giving specific pastoral responses are central to this study. Under these two themes, mainline mission churches and Pentecostal-Charismatic churches, which describe themselves as evangelical, have been identified as 'E-churches', to distinguish them from other churches such as the *sunsum sɔre* (spiritual churches) and neo-prophetic churches.[15]

a. *Help-seeking from multiple sources*

The collected data indicates that all the women respondents went to several places (at least three) for help. Most of them sought help not just from their own church family, but from several Christian churches and prayer centres of different kinds. Here is a typical extract from the interviews:

> ...Accra Psychiatric Hospital; then from the hospital to my church, the Church of Pentecost in Mamprobi. From there I think I was also sent to a herbalist at Odorkor Kwashieman... Then I went to All Nations Church Ministry International... And from there to the Bible Based Ministry... Any other church you hear of, you go and I think Edumfa Prayer Camp... Yes, many. I went to the Church of [the Lord,] Aladura, where I stayed long...(Kaaley)

Irrespective of the above account, most of the women employed Christian spiritual resources (that is, primarily prayer, counselling and sometimes deliverance sessions) from churches that are deemed evangelical in outlook/ tradition (E-churches). From the data, though, only two of the women respondents (20%) sought help from only *one* E-church. The same two also used other resources like the hospital and herbal-based medicine. One respondent, although a member of an E-church, did not ask her church for help because she felt they did not care. Instead, she sought help from other places. Adjo, Respondent 4, did not seek help from any church or pastor (E-church or otherwise) because she had experienced some stigma and shame from her own E-church because of her unmarried status:

> How do I go to such a person for counselling if being divorced is already creating problems without him telling me you asked for it? I would not consider going to a pastor, in fact, this had made me very cynical towards pastors.

b. *Help-seeking from formal mental health institutions/ practitioners.*

It is noteworthy, however, that every one of them sought the services of professional mental health practitioners at some point in the course of their ailment, in addition to using spiritual resources. There were mixed responses about the use of mental health facilities and practitioners, concerning the attitudes, treatment and help received. Amma had this to say about a public health facility:

So she [the nurse] took a cane and will cane you and make you feel as if you are so useless and hopeless in this world...

Thankfully, it appears the facility eventually took steps to improve its services:
The third time, it wasn't so bad and I think because of that, I didn't have a problem walking into the ... Hospital anymore because I felt that it wasn't a bad place. It's friendlier now. (Amma)

However, another respondent had a more positive experience at the same facility on her first visit:
But in the first time...because I was called Doctor, I had a wonderful time. It was also at that time that that fear of great trouble was leaving me because I was on medication, so I felt freer. (Akua)

On her part, Rita, was able to separate her experiences with the professional mental health practitioners at the same facility from her experience as an in-patient:
The psychiatrists themselves have patience and time for you, but it's just the treatment given to you in the boarding facility [which] is not good.

Not all the women used the public facility mentioned above. However, they shared their experience of how they were handled by the mental health professionals at the different facilities. Respondents 4 and 5 reported it thus:

[W]e started well but his approach made me feel worse. I would come back from the consultation feeling worse than I felt when I went in... (Adjo)

I can say she (clinical psychologist) is a very high-class person, (but) she understood me, had patience with me and she talked to me nicely... (Bema)

Interestingly, three (30%) of the women narrated that they came across professional practitioners who integrated their Christian faith into their practice:
With the psychologists and psychiatrists, they came from the medicine angle. Those who were Christians added their faith; those who were not did not... (Naki)

...[t]he lady combines both pastoral and clinical skills. So I am still with her...she's been there for me... (Adjo)

Indeed, Kaaley, stated that a psychiatrist told her he thought her issue was more of 'a spiritual thing' because her issue was 'so different'. These narratives are significant because after several years of hostility between psychological practice and Christian theology, many in the West are working actively towards integrating religion, spirituality and faith into their practice.[16] It appears, though, that in Ghana, there is not much of a debate about professionals integrating spirituality into their practice. It is possible that it has been taken for granted because of the Ghanaian religio-cultural context and primal consciousness. This implies that it may not be problematic for practitioners to integrate their faith into their work and respond more effectively to some of the spiritual issues and yearnings arising from the condition of their patients. Interestingly, in my interview with Chief Psychiatrist Dr Akwasi Osei, he said younger doctors hardly tolerate the inclusion of spiritual beliefs in the requests of patients, but as an experienced doctor, he does. According to him,

> I do not work against a person's beliefs; I work around it... I try to convince them that taking their medication is not incompatible with their beliefs.[17]

It is significant, though, that nine (90%) of the women reported that they started getting well or saw a reduction in symptoms, or gained better understanding of their condition when they consulted professional mental health practitioners, even though at the time of their interviews, seven (70%) respondents had not experienced full recovery, as captured by some of the extracts below:

> I am feeling much better now...I think my mother saw it so I was given medication early so it didn't become as bad as it usually is...(Amma)

> [Clinical psychologist], knew her stuff, she was a very seasoned psychologist because then, she knew what was wrong with me and then that was the beginning of my recovery... (Naki)

> ...[w]hen I started taking the medication, it helped me. It really did and I was also able to control my diet effectively... (Adjo)

One can infer from their responses that although medication was helpful, it was limited in providing complete recovery or healing, since almost all the women were at various levels of recovery: some were still experiencing relapses, while others were managing their situations; but for the majority, the medication made them functional again. Others found much relief in the individual counselling they received and, for Korkor, Respondent 6, a support group proved to be quite helpful:

> When I came to the support group, I saw and heard a lot of stories about people with OCD, and I saw after all I am not the only one in this condition. I was very much encouraged that something can be done... and I saw that there is hope for me.

c. *Help-seeking from herbal medicine and other religious resources*
Apart from the medication prescribed by the hospital, Respondent 9, Efua, also relied heavily on herbal medicine to cure her brain tumour, which appeared to be the primary cause of her mental illness. This medicine, supplied by a foreign-owned Ghanaian company, appeared to have brought her the positive results that Western medicine could not achieve.

> I saw the BasicNeeds treatment as a way of helping me manage my mental problem but the Herbal School helped me cure it completely. (Efua)

Two respondents used the services of a number of *sunsum sɔre* who, in addition to prayer and fasting, employed 'florida water'[18] and herbal concoctions, which the women described as 'painful' treatments. As Kaaley narrated,

> [I]t is herbal. They called it 'devil's incense' and it was very painful; it had a stench. It's not easy and you had to go every morning...

These women eventually went back to using the medical/mental health resources (medicine and therapy), while one returned to an E-church for further help. Two respondents, Korkor and Kaaley consulted neo-prophetic pastors in addition to other resources. Whereas one of the so-called prophets defrauded the family of Korkor, Kaaley was asked to sleep with the prophet she saw, for exorcism, but she refused. These are excerpts of their narrations

> My mother was desperate...So my mother went to give the money to the prophet. And ever since, the prophet has not called my mother again. When you call him, he has switched off his phone   (Korkor)

> [A]s the man of God claim (sic), 'I have to bathe you naked for seven days; you have to come and stay in my room and I will have to sleep with you so that I can suck the spiritual husband from you...' (Kaaley)

I discovered that family members of the respondents who sought help from traditional shrines and neo-prophetic churches actually sent them there, seemingly, against their will. Some of the non-Christian sources included a Buddhist temple,[19] traditional shrines[20] and a traditional herbalist.[21]

Respondent 2, Akua, visited a number of E-churches for fellowship and prayer, but did not ask them directly for help for fear of being stigmatised:

> I didn't trust anybody in the church enough to let them know about how I feel because I had known enough about the stigma around and all that so I wouldn't go to church and tell.

It emerged in the interview, however, that in her youth, Akua had been taken to several traditional shrines for help, although her father was a leader in a Charismatic church:

> [F]rom Accra Psychiatric Hospital, I went to Akonedi Shrine in Larteh. From there, I went to Nana Atia Nframa at Akweti Junction on the Afete road. From there I came home but I didn't know where they came [from], but spiritualists came to the house to take care of me, fetish priests and all, I mean... (Akua)

d. Help-seeking from Prayer Centres and Camps

Those respondents who reported that they went to prayer centres for help had different experiences. Some were good and helpful in their treatment, while others were largely negative experiences. For instance, Amma reported receiving cruel treatment in a camp run by a prophet:

> ...[b]ut when I think of the physical conditions I was put under in M (the camp), it makes me cringe. I didn't like the environment; we were chained to the floor. We were treated like animals and even though there was a partition between the males and females, when the females were walking out, we saw all these naked males making suggestive gestures at you, shouting things at you; and where the ladies took their bath was in the view of the men. It wasn't a nice place to be. When I compare it to B (another camp), B was like a heaven and M wasn't good at all...

Interestingly, the respondents narrated that some of the Christian prayer centres they used were established by persons and churches connected with the evangelical tradition (such as Patmos Christian Centre, Akropong, and Boka camp set up by a Church of Pentecost member). In such places, in contrast, the respondents reported pleasant experiences:

> [T]he environment (Patmos) was very nice, pleasant, neat and quiet. There is soothing music played there throughout the day and you are given free range; there is a library for you to look at the books, there are people who are nice to you, the prayer meetings too are nice and very engaging. (Amma)

> When I went to Boka, the woman was very friendly...we just go in for prayers there. She talked to you nicely, giving you promises of God that it will be well. (Bema)

Others were not clearly defined as associated with any particular Christian tradition, but more of the neo-prophetic and *sunsum sɔre* kind. The cruelty Amma experienced is echoed in the experience of Akua, in a *sunsum sɔre* camp in Kumasi:

> I was chained. I was beaten. I was insulted, and that is where my faith was really shaken. If these people claim that they are really for God, why all this?

However, Akua's experience at a traditional shrine was pleasant in contrast:

> I was the only one who could go and sit at her (traditional priest) feet and talk to her the whole time...Very welcoming... it's only that it was idol worship that is why I didn't want to go there.

Thus, it is important to note that seeking help from multiple places and resources for mental distress/illness is not a peculiar thing, because of the nature of the condition, the persistence of symptoms in most cases and the desperation to gain a sense of freedom and wellbeing. Furthermore, all the respondents affirmed that, when it comes to mental health issues, women are more likely than men to seek help not only for their own wellbeing, but also because of the central role they play to sustain their families.[22] The respondents also believed that their own condition invariably affects their families' health and sought to do everything to alleviate it, as illustrated in the following comments:

> I would oversleep. I couldn't bathe my daughter; I couldn't even breast-feed her. A baby around four months...I told them to reduce the dosage for me so I could take care of my daughter and they did... (Rita)

> Last night, my son looked at me and said you are not caring and it cut deep because he wasn't feeling well. And my son could not understand that I was not well...that I can't get up from my bed, get to the shower and put on a dress and drive him to the hospital [crying] ... (Adjo)

Experiences with Specific Pastoral Responses from EGPs

It has been established that the majority (80%) of the women respondents I interviewed sought help from evangelical pastors and churches (E-churches).[23] Some of the women narrated both pleasant and helpful experiences. Two examples of the positive experiences are captured below:

> ...[t]he pastor would pray for you. But they will make you understand that once you have God's Word in you, it wasn't a demonic thing. 'So use the word of God to battle whatever problems you are going through.' And that helped me a lot. (Amma)

> [H]e [the pastor] was perfect. I mean he wasn't partial in anything. He was there for everybody. His doctrine was to meet the spiritual aspect of the person. (Rita)

Some respondents had largely negative experiences at the E-churches visited:

> ...[t]he church ... they will just come and be speaking in tongues and be doing their thing for you and they go. Nobody cares about your welfare until there is anything more alarming... (Kaaley)

> They didn't do anything. Eventually, they gave me some of the salt to take home that was when I realised they had used me. (Rita)

> You tell them and they say ...we don't see what is troubling you. I was thinking that they were joking with me, but what I told them it's no joke. If it were not troubling me, I would not have told them. They don't really see it [as] a problem. (Naki)

Some respondents felt stigmatised and even insulted by some of the responses they received:

> With ... (E-church), because I was not working and not in the university, it was like I was ignored ... (Korkor)

> [H]e [the pastor] wasn't sincere with me in the sense that when he was referring me to the prayer warriors, I saw him make this sign [pointing her index finger to the side of her head repeatedly] ... meaning this person is mad. (Naki)

Naki relates another harrowing experience with another pastor:

> [W]hen I went, I was so ill or possessed or whatever was happening to me, I couldn't even sit down to listen to anything. So he said we should

pray and of course I couldn't pray so he told me that you only find flies at the garbage dump; then I understood what he was trying to tell me. That if I have become garbage, that is why the spirit... whatever.

However, she had a more pleasant experience with another EGP:
He [the pastor] prayed with me and assured me. I said I feel I am possessed and he said a Christian doesn't get possessed. I left there feeling happy but by the time I got home, I was back to square one. (Naki)

Abraham A. Berinyuu,[24] Esther Acolatse,[25] Sarah-Louise Hurst[26] and several others have stressed the critical role clergy play in responding to mental distress. This was confirmed by the help-seeking behaviour of the women survivors I interviewed.

Collaboration between EGPs and Professional Mental Health Practitioners

The EGPs the women saw gave primarily spiritual explanations for their distress and prescribed primarily spiritual solutions. Indeed, the data shows that only two (20%) of the respondents mentioned that the EGPs they consulted suggested they continue to see their professional MHPs and take their medication. The EGPs' focus on the spiritual was reflected in some of the women's responses:

Prayer [is] spiritual, so they don't say anything about the mental hospital or anything... (Kaaley)

The experience was not bad but they also didn't recommend hospital. Maybe it's because when I talk, I sound very intelligent. (Naki)

However, from the analysis, the EGPs seen by the women respondents appeared to listen to them and make some sort of assessment as illustrated below from some of the women's stories:

[H]e just prayed for me and also assured me that it is no more part of me. It is the demons that were doing that and they are no more part of me. (Naki)

This [E-church] went to [an] extreme dimension... like 'Maame Water' spirit used me to do something, but with [another E-church], they said I am a very bright girl and the demons want to torment my mind so that I won't be useful. (Korkor)

While one (EGP) thought I was going off, the other (EGP of another church) felt that something in our family was chasing us to disgrace ourselves, working against the women... (Naki)

The content and depth of assessment of the treatment are difficult to tell. The above extracts indicate that different EGPs sometimes reached different conclusions on causality on the same case. For methods of response, the data shows that the EGPs primarily used prayer, sharing Scripture verses and teaching the respondents to declare such over their lives, encouragement from the Scriptures and deliverance/exorcism. A few EGPs encouraged the respondents to fast. Unlike those women who also received help from *sunsum sɔre* leaders, including baths, application of 'florida water' and other scents, oils, prolonged fasting and exorcism/deliverance exercises, the respondents who consulted EGPs hardly mentioned them using such items and practices. That does not however suggest that such items were never used. In fact, Efua, (Respondent 9) mentioned that the EGP gave her salt for bathing. A few respondents also mentioned the use of church rituals. For instance, one was served Holy Communion by her priest, while in another case, the EGP gave the respondent wine to drink:

The pastor received me; prayed for me then they gave me something to drink. It was like a wine... That wine saved my life that night. (Efua)

Since the EGPs appeared to undertake their own methods of assessment, assigned causality and proceeded to provide the response which best matched their assessment, this may explain why only a couple of the EGPs the women consulted suggested they see a mental health practitioner. In effect, most EGPs did not see the reason to refer them to one.

Perception of the Knowledge base of EGPs

Five (50%) of the women respondents firmly believed that the EGPs were quite ignorant when it came to emotional/mental distress or illness:

[The pastor]... didn't know what was wrong with me. They thought that by praying, whatever is worrying you is stopped. (Efua)

If you think somebody with bipolar is the same as somebody with a broken heart, you are not handling it properly. They don't even know what it is so if you go to a pastor and say I have a bipolar problem, he will say what is that? (Amma)

I stopped going because I didn't think it was addressing what was going on inside me. [Pastor] was compassionate but he never said I should get to the hospital or anything, he felt that if he prayed for me... (Naki)

[O]ur pastors are clueless when it comes to psychosomatic diseases. Because they tend to see it as a weakness of faith and that for a sufferer of depression is painful. (Adjo)

I also educated him. I don't know whether he went to research through, that one I don't know. So based on how I explained the OCD, he saw that it was difficult. He went to explain to the senior pastor that there is somebody going through this and it's strange... (Korkor)

The perception that a pastoral responder is ignorant is bound to affect the impact he/she makes on the help-seeker; the likely result is diminished hope for a solution. It is difficult to tell whether the appreciable educational level of majority of the women had anything to do with this perception. However, they made recommendations to address this perceived ignorance.

Recommendations for EGPs and Churches

As a result of their experiences, seven (70%) of the women respondents insisted that E-churches and pastors should go beyond spiritual prescriptions and be educated on mental health issues. The two extracts below illustrate the struggle that Christian sufferers face when confronted with the interplay of suspicion between psychology and Christianity in their pastoral caregivers. They considered that this lack of trust may actually undermine the sufferer's quest for healing:

They need a bit of knowledge themselves. They always struggle between spiritual and medicine, as for that one, they always struggle. When is it maybe spiritual? When do we bring or allow them to go for medication? Because even me as a Christian suffering the condition, it was something I used to battle with until I got to the point where I saw myself being destroyed and so I stopped worrying about the spiritual aspect and yearned for medication... (Naki)

The kind of pastor who understands and knows what is really wrong with the person; because with an educated mind you will read and find out what is really wrong. But with these uneducated pastors shouting around, you wouldn't know what the outcome would be; we don't... (Serwa)

They also believed that the EGPs needed to work hand in hand with professional mental health practitioners, as captured in this extract:

> I think that they should not only look at it as the spiritual; there is a belief that the devil is behind every sickness; sickness is spirit but for them to actually get to the root of the problem with the mental illnesses... you can't just deal with it at the spiritual level and leave it there. So I think if they can work hand in hand with the medical experts, then I think it will be easier and the patients can also recover very fast because if you put it in the patient's mind that it's a demon, that is Ghana mentality. (Korkor)

Personal Faith and Spirituality and Coping with Emotional/Mental Distress

Faith and spirituality presented strength and hope for the women in their condition. Two of the women describe how they applied these in their helpless moments:

> People can do whatever, but you have to draw the strength from within you and usually you can't find it from people that much. They may want to do everything but you have to reach out to a force above you. A force like that, for me, is God. And Scripture has been a wonderful, wonderful opportunity... (Adjo)

> The Bible says that faith cometh by hearing and hearing the Word of God. So, I believe that I have not given up. I still... even though I am going through medical treatment, I know that one day God will touch me and I will not see the OCD again in my mind. That will be total healing. And if there is going to be a testimony, it has not yet happened, but I believe that my faith has increased based on me hearing the things God can do. (Korkor)

At the same time, faith and spirituality raised some puzzling questions, and some of the respondents found their faith incongruous to their health conditions. This is the case with many Christians who have suffered similar illnesses:

> It just happens that I could be a Christian and have a disease; and nobody will associate it with demons. So why is it that when am a Christian and I have a mental problem, it is associated with demons all the time? ... I remember one day, the pastor said that how can Jesus be living in you and demons be living in you at the same time? And it hit me, and it's true, we are vessels; we are God's temple. Jesus is living in us; so when we take Jesus as our personal Saviour, he comes

to live in us, the Holy Spirit lives in us. So, how come the Holy Spirit will be living in the same temple as demons? It doesn't quite work, and I took a cue from that...(Amma)

I told myself that I was going to live the best way I knew until one day, I dropped dead or something. I used to pray that God should have mercy on me many times and quote the scriptures but it didn't remove the underlying thing within me that I was beyond redemption. So I was being like how a Christian is supposed to be, always praying to God to have mercy on me. (Naki)

Rita, expressed her feelings in song during the interview:

There is only one hymn I ask them to pray with; [singing] 'Good Lord, remember, oh Thou from who (sic) all blessing flow, I lift my heart for Thee, He clears my sorrows and all my woes. Good Lord, remember me. Good Lord, remember me. Good Lord, remember me, because the work that I have to do for God, I am not able to do it.'

Ultimately for the women, it is the incarnate God who can truly and completely heal them from their mental distresses, however He chooses to do so. This is expressed in various ways, and succinctly summed up by Rita in this extract:

God says we should all bring our problems to him. That is why he died on the cross for us. It is not a person who will save us; it is God himself who has come as a person, who has used his grace and his blood to save us, that is what our belief is in.

Suffice it to say that the data collected from the ten Christian women survivors was rich and filled with real human emotion, wisdom and surprising strength of mind and purpose. In their struggles with selfhood and self-understanding in the face of serious affliction, and their struggles with help-seeking, societal and self-stigma notwithstanding, they all still held on to the Christian hope of trust in a faithful, loving and sovereign God. All of them believed that God is able to deliver them from their suffering. No matter how incongruous they thought their mental condition was in relation to their Christian faith, they demonstrated resilience and perseverance by holding on in faith to Jesus Christ as their Saviour and their Healer. In so doing, they reflected the tenacious faith seen not only in the likes of Charles H. Spurgeon,[27] Martin Luther[28] and John Bunyan,[29] themselves men survivors of bygone centuries, but also in people like authors Chonda Pierce,[30] Kathryn Greene-McCreight[31] and Cathy Wield,[32] the women survivors of modern times.

In the view of Andrew F. Walls, the ten women respondents were theologising in their specific agonising contexts, attempting to 'think in a Christian way'. Also, the need for the choices and decisions they made, or which were made on their behalf, arose 'from specific settings in life'.[33] Even though some had personally struggled with the use of Western medicine, seeing it as a sort of weakness, their recommendations to the EGPs and pastors actively demonstrated what they believed to be the best approach, that is, a careful 'marriage' or integration of the benefits of the science of psychotherapy and medicine with faith and spirituality, in a way that brings honour to God and upholds Him as Lord over all things.

It is important to note here how the weaknesses and strengths in Ghana's formal mental health system, as well as those in the complementary and alternative systems, emerged from the information the women gave me. Issues raised earlier in the study, including stigma, discrimination, effects of child abuse and violence against women, human rights violations, the impact of women's multiple roles as well as the socio-cultural and religious African worldview all emerged as issues of import from the women's interviews. This affirms indeed, that first-line and other responders, including pastors, reflect their religious and cultural milieu when confronted with such conditions. This matter is further affirmed by the information I garnered from the interviews with Evangelical Ghanaian Pastors.

CHAPTER SEVEN

PASTORS RESPONDING: PERCEPTIONS ON SYMPTOMS, GENDER DIFFERENCES AND CAUSES

Introduction

Pastors from churches which identify as evangelical, who for the purposes of this study, I describe as Evangelical Ghanaian Pastors (EGPs) are the study's primary respondents. The preceding chapter, which details Ghanaian Christian women's experiences present complementary and contrasting data to what was obtained from the EGPs.

The EGPs were selected from four church denominations in Ghana. These are the Presbyterian Church of Ghana (PCG), Church of Pentecost, Ghana (COP), Assemblies of God, Ghana (AOG) and the International Central Gospel Church (ICGC).[1] All the denominations have branches spread across the country. Working across that range of denominations increased the likelihood of capturing the general tenor of thought, experiences and perceptions of these pastors regarding mental health and women's mental health issues in particular.

The headquarters of each denomination made available to me the names of all the senior pastors of their branch churches in the five districts selected for the study. These districts are the Accra Metropolitan District, Ho Municipal District, Kumasi Metropolitan District, Tamale Metropolitan District, and Wa Municipal District. In those five districts and in each of the four denominations, one pastor was randomly selected out of each set of names from the different denominations. In other words, five pastors were interviewed in each district. Thus, I interviewed a total of twenty pastors from the four denominations across the selected five districts in Ghana.

The biographical profile of the EGPs was quite interesting. Most of the EGPs turned out to be in their fifties, the mean age being 50.25 years. All but one (5%) was married, with the exception being also the youngest. Their educational backgrounds ranged from the senior secondary school to the postgraduate degree levels: five (25%) did not hold any university degree or its equivalent, even though they were all formally educated, some at diploma and certificate levels. While six (30%) EGPs had a graduate degree or its equivalent, eight (35%) held postgraduate degrees, mostly Master's degrees, and one (5%) had a doctorate. All had been educated at one theological institution or the other in the country, most having been trained at the theological institutions established by their various denominations. In the Table below, the EGPs have been assigned numerical identities (1, 2, 3...) in the order in which they were interviewed. I also assigned them pseudo names prefixed by the short form of the title Reverend (Rev.), since they are all ordained clergy.

Table 2: Profile of EGP Respondents

Respondent	Age	Marital Status	Educational level	Ethnic Affiliation	Sex
1 (Rev Nanor)	52	Married	Graduate	Ada (Dangbe)	Male
2 (Rev Mawu)	57	Married	Postgraduate	Keta (Ewe)	Male
3 (Rev Doku)	50	Married	Below first degree	Dzodze (Ewe)	Male
4 (Rev Anan)	42	Married	Postgraduate	Akropong-Akuapem (Akan)	Male
5 (Rev Prah)	52	Married	Graduate	Senya Brentuo (Akan)	Male
6 (Rev Akyia)	58	Married	Postgraduate	Larteh-Akuapem (Guan)	Male
7 (Rev Bia)	56	Married	Postgraduate	Dawu-Akuapem (Guan)	Male
8 (Rev Quao)	54	Married	Postgraduate	Teshie (Ga)	Male
9 (Rev Atta)	55	Married	Below first degree	Cape Coast (Akan)	Male
10 (Rev Ntow)	39	Married	Graduate level	Aburi-Akuapem (Akan)	Male
11 (Rev Osei)	57	Married	Below first degree	Apromase-Ejisu (Akan)	Male
12 (Rev Poku)	49	Married	Postgraduate	Asokore-Asante (Akan)	Male
13 (Rev Suni)	51	Married	Graduate	Nandom (Dagaare)	Male

14 (Rev Onua)	57	Married	Postgraduate	Larteh-Akuapem (Guan)	Male
15 Rev Awuni)	47	Married	Graduate	Tongo (Talensi)	Male
16 (Rev Bona)	59	Married	Below first degree	Bodada (Ewe)	Male
17 (Rev Nsiah)	42	Married	Below first degree	Nsuta-Kwaman (Akan)	Male
18 (Rev Tuuli)	27	Single	Graduate	Nadowli (Dagaare)	Male
19 (Rev Naa-ba)	53	Married	Postgraduate	Garu (Kusaali)	Male
20 (Rev Dua)	48	Married	Graduate	Anyan Abaasa (Akan)	Male

It must be noted, however, that because most pastors of church denominations are male (particularly in the COP, which has an exclusively male pastorate), no female pastor emerged out of the random sampling process.

A total of eleven (11) main themes emerged based on the research questions administered to the EGPs. Each theme had a number of sub-themes. The main themes were discussed with illustrative extracts or quotes from the responses, followed by my interpretation of the emerging patterns, recurring themes and sub-themes. This chapter presents the first four of the major themes, while the other seven are presented in the following chapter.

Evangelical Ghanaian Pastors' (EGPs) Views and Perceptions on Symptoms, Gender Differences and Causes of Emotional or Mental Distress and Illness
Under this broad heading, the following four (4) themes emerged, namely, the EGPs' personal experience of mental/emotional health difficulties in friends, family or congregants; observable symptoms and perceived manifestations of emotional distress/mental illness; perceptions of gender differences in presenting symptoms; and perceived causes of emotional distress/mental illness.

a. *EGPs Personal Experience of Emotional/Mental Health Difficulties in Friends, Family or Congregants*
Six (30%) of the EGPs had the experience of seeing family members and persons close to them affected by mental health challenges. There were different reactions to the situations. Some found them rather disturbing, and felt especially uneasy with the stigma. The experiences of three of the EGPs are captured below:

...[a] nephew, way back more than twenty years ago... It was really disturbing because these things, especially in our cultural setting, the way people look at this without looking at the other side, that scientifically it is a kind of sickness like any other sickness, but it has stigma and things so it was really disturbing. *(Rev Akyia)*

I think one of my sister's children... When she was born, according to my parents, in the course of birth she fell but I don't know what happened. She grew up with a mental disability... It hasn't been very easy because as a pastor, I have a lot of friends and when we go home she starts behaving in some strange ways. I had to educate my friends on her condition. *(Rev Awuni)*

He is a first cousin. He was travelling to Asentrewa. On the way, at a crossroad, he saw mashed yam with egg on the road. He took it and ate, and since then, that has been the case...We felt embittered because this sickness was not from childhood. *(Rev Nsiah).*

The stigma of mental illness is real. Nor does it pertain only to Africa or African Christians. Cathy Wield recalls her own experience: 'I attended a conference on "Christians, the Bible and Psychology" in London in 2010. The question was put to the floor as to whether there was more stigma within the churches or outside in the world and sadly an overwhelming majority voted "within the churches".[2] The responses of the EGPs show that they were neither immune to societal stigma on their families when a member was mentally challenged, nor indifferent in their own personal feelings. One EGP had the painful experience of observing mental illness in his wife:

It was my wife...I felt empathy for her. I prayed the Lord to intervene... she can't stay alone in the house and anywhere I am going, she has to follow me...for the past six years. *(Rev Bia)*

b. *Observable Symptoms and Perceived Manifestations of Emotional/ Mental Distress or Illness*

This theme was identified from the perspective of the EGP respondents as they described the symptoms observed in people with mental/emotional distress or illness. It includes symptoms they had seen exhibited by people with mental/emotional distress or illness, many of whom were congregants or persons they had ministered to; and those symptoms they perceived in such people as well. The sub-themes employed in explaining the major theme are: Bizarre behaviours (or perceived manifestations); Emotional displays and Physiological symptoms.

i. Bizarre Behaviours

All the EGPs reported observing the awkward and bizarre behaviours of affected persons manifestly different from their normal behaviours. Some of the unusual behaviours involved self-harm, while others appeared to be connected with religious activity or belief. Below are some instances of observed bizarre behaviours as narrated by the respondents:

> It all started when she went to the market one day and came back with anchovies – 'momoni' in her brassier...*(Rev Nanor)*

> She is tossing herself around and wants to strip herself naked and everybody is running away from her... *(Rev Naaba)*

> He was at times just indoors, not allowing anybody to come to talk to him at all. There was a time his mother said he even tried castrating himself and that was disturbing... one time we were dealing with him and he started doing press ups. He almost at one time clubbed the deacon with a pestle. They had to really whisk him away. *(Rev Akyia)*

> When she sees me, she just approaches and hugs me and wants to kiss me. She will tell me, 'Pastor, you look so handsome'. Then she will sometimes tell me that we will be getting married, so I should fix the date for her. *(Rev Bia)*

Descriptions of symptoms of bizarre behaviours seemingly connected with the sufferers' religious action or belief are highlighted below:

> When she was a child, a fetish priest worked on her and since then she has not been ok. She came to the church to be prayed for. She can't sit at one place. She will come to you and after talking to her she will go and come back to you over and over [again]. *(Rev Nsiah)*

> One case was of a person who was very prayerful. He was going into the forest and praying and he spent months praying... One day, all of a sudden on that day it was raining and instead of him leaving the place and coming home he decided to stay there. The family called to find out and he would tell them I took some people and we went to the forest in a vehicle and put him in. I knew that there was a problem... *(Rev Dua)*

As witnessed by the EGPs, bizarre behaviour accompanied by religious belief or action raises the question of religion as a possible factor in mental illness. Kate Loewenthal extensively discusses some psychiatrists' belief that religion itself is problematic because it contributes to or complicates mental illness.[3] Harold Koenig however demonstrates in his research that, generally speaking, religious belief is a strong factor in both the prevention of mental ill-health and coping with such conditions.[4] Because African Christians, particularly women, are very much engaged in high levels of religious activities, I believe that it is important for professionals and pastoral caregivers to discern whether religious activity itself contributes to a sufferer's condition or the condition is distinct from religious activity. This would help to craft an appropriate response to the sufferer. One EGP account affirms the need for such discernment:

> ...[a]nother church member, a young man [he] fell from a height and within that week; nothing happened so everybody thought he was ok, then he entered into fasting which of course I warned him about... He went into it and then his 'head became bigger'...As a spiritual father, definitely you will feel so bad and sorry for them. For the young man, I sort of blame him for being disobedient...
> (Rev Nanor)

ii. Emotional displays
Some EGPs were able to deduce the conditions of mental illness/emotional distress from the emotional displays they observed:

> When she gave birth... we were going to the hospital and she didn't want me to hold the baby. That was the symptom I saw initially. She was also crippled with fear... *(Rev Bia)*

> It was a guy who was mentioning the name of a girl continuously that he loved that girl. The case was that the girl... broke off with him, and he was mentally disturbed. *(Rev Ntow)*

iii. Physiological symptoms
Some of the respondents recounted observing behaviours best captured as physiological symptoms, which may or may not accompany emotional displays:

> She can't sit at one place, and when she talks, the words are not clear and meaningful... *(Rev Nsiah)*

> ...[a]nd you see the person not moving at all... *(Rev Suni)*

The lady was growing lean and at a point some members of the congregation thought she was going mad. She sometimes talks and other times is quiet; other times it is as if she is hearing strange voices. Sometimes I will greet her and she wouldn't respond... *(Rev Awuni)*

The various descriptions the EGPs gave of observed symptoms no doubt attest to their familiarity with cases of emotional/mental distress or illness in their work as ministers. It was therefore surprising when asked about formal categories of mental illnesses, that almost all of them (95%) could not name even the commonest of mental diseases, such as depression or anxiety. Joseph Ciarrocchi's statement that '...knowledge of abnormal psychology, the science of mental illness, is essential for ministry,'[5] could very well apply to the EGP respondents in this study.

iv. Perceptions of Gender Differences in Presenting Symptoms

To better understand the approaches of the EGPs in their response to cases of emotional distress/mental illness and to women sufferers in particular, I asked about their perceptions of the differences they saw in the presenting symptoms between men and women. This was an important question because their underlying assumptions about gendered manifestations of these conditions could also provide a clue about their choice of approaches in interventions. Their answers were clustered into the following sub-themed statements: Women are more prone to mental illness and distress than men; Women exhibit more mental illness and distress symptoms than men; Women and men exhibit different mental illness and distress symptoms; and, Women are gullible, more trusting and emotionally weaker than men. I now examine each of the statements.

i. Women are more prone to mental illness and distress than men

Ten EGPs (50%) perceived women as being more vulnerable to emotional distress and mental illness, thus affirming global data. The WHO reports roughly equal rates of mental illness between women and men, but notes that women have much higher rates of depression, anxiety and unipolar disorders.[6] The reasons the EGPs gave for their perceptions were however definitely gendered, as illustrated in the two responses below:

...[i]n fact, most at times, it is the women who go through these kinds of problems. With my personal experience, I will say about 85% goes to the women and 15% to the men... *(Rev Quao)*

I think that women by nature are emotional. Then, they don't hide emotional circumstances, so anything [that] disturbs [them], the little things make some women just, should I say, 'go off'. *(Rev Akyia)*

ii. Women exhibit more mental illness and distress symptoms than men
Following their perception that women are more prone to mental illness, four (20%) EGPs believed that women exhibit more symptoms of mental illness and distress than men. This view also correlates with their perception that women are more expressive when distressed, as illustrated below:

...[b]ecause theirs is often times more visible than that of men...
(Rev Osei)

...[s]ince women are more vocal about it, we see theirs more than men...
(Rev Mawu)

...[a]nd the woman has all her heart in the man, the reaction is sometimes so violent and spontaneous that she falls into something else.
(Rev Naaba)

iii. Women and men exhibit different mental illness and distress symptoms
Fifteen (75%) of the EGPs were of the view that women and men exhibit different symptoms of mental illness and distress. Some of the interesting perceptions are shared below where the EGPs compared and contrasted, for example, talkativeness in women as against stoic behaviour in men, or aggressiveness and violence in men, which is largely absent in women. Many of their views fit into the society's gendered perceptions of behaviour, even among the mentally sound:

The women are calm and the men are sometimes aggressive. The women are also neater compared to the men... *(Rev Bia)*

I see that [in] most of the ladies in the church who have this kind of problem, during worship, some will climb the platform to try to sing with the choir, something you don't usually see among the men who have this kind of problem. The man will be quiet and rather go out, but the woman would want to participate. *(Rev Poku)*

Some EGPs felt that men's sense of pride and stubbornness keeps them from being expressive about their distress:

Women are easily disturbed. And when they are disturbed, you can easily see it. But men try to be stubborn. Men may have problems but because of pride and stubbornness, they try to hide it but women are easily disturbed. *(Rev Prah)*

For men, it is difficult to voice it out when he is going through difficulties or stress but women would always want to voice it out. Women believe that the more they voice things out, they will get solutions. While men too believe that as long as I keep the thing within me, I will find a way out. *(Rev Mawu)*

With men, they tend to harbour it inside. So even though it's eating them up, they try to prove strong, probably until they are pushed to the wall before they can [talk]. Another difference with the men is that, because they try to harbour it, by the time it comes out, it can be more serious than that of the women. *(Rev Osei)*

Ebenezer Abboah-Offei and Theresa Wiafe-Asante, the Christian deliverance practitioners I interviewed, both told me they see more women than men in their work, and that the men 'want to handle it themselves'[7] and 'they often try to solve their own problems, and if they can't, then they seek help...which takes more work.'[8] The implication of such gendered behaviour is that for men, the likelihood that emotional and mental illness is underreported is real. This presents a danger because distress often escalates when left untreated. More research is needed in Ghana in the area of men's behaviour in times of emotional or mental difficulties. Also, the situation urgently calls for studies specific to Christian men in distress.

iv. Women are gullible, more trusting, and emotionally weaker than men
Nine (45%) of the EGP respondents generally held the view that women go through these experiences because they are more trusting, more gullible and emotionally weaker than men. These views largely affirm the findings of the research by Angela Ofori-Atta and her colleagues[9] on how the public perceive women with mental illness.

While three EGPs (15%) used the word 'weak' to describe women emotionally, two (10%) of them actually used Scripture to justify that perception:

They are weak vessels. When the Bible says they are weak vessels, it is talking about their emotional strength. They usually need support, security and when they are losing these things they begin to fear and that fear causes them to come out with a lot of expressions...

(Rev Poku)
I think it's how they were created. The Bible says [they] are weaker vessels and they think a lot about things. Things they consider most important, we the men brush over it (sic). For instance, if someone promised to marry a man, and it fails, then men will not worry about it. Women could have broken hearts as a result and it will bring a lot of emotional distress. *(Rev Nsiah)*

Most women are weak emotionally, so as soon as they are disturbed, you will see that their facial expression changes, they become dejected. *(Rev Osei)*

Those who believed women are equally too trusting and gullible explained why:
...[m]aybe their physiological make-up, maybe too their upbringing and the way they were groomed, and sometimes they believe people so easily...*(Rev Anan)*

The saying goes [that] men use their brains to do things and women use their hearts. I think that is one of the major factors that affect them [more] emotionally than men. Once they like something, their heart goes out; they don't think about the consequence of it...*(Rev Tuuli)*

[A] woman, especially a married woman, when she accepts you as her man, hardly will you hear that she is cheating on her husband... Women believe what they hear, so when they come to trust a man, he can be lying; but so far as they are not a factor of the lies, they believe him. When they later on find out that what they believe was a lie, it really upsets them a lot...*(Rev Awuni)*

When a woman wants to do something, she does it with her heart. So when disappointments or failures come, it (sic) brings about some challenges, which she can't bear. That results in those things...*(Rev Bia)*

Some EGPs felt that women tend to overreact to issues, an indication of their inability to deal with life's stresses:
Sometimes they are not able to cope with things men see as simple and overlook. But the women's reaction can carry them to a point where they will need support. So that is the kind of cases that we see. They react beyond measure and then they will have to come for counselling. *(Rev Naaba)*

Women are very vulnerable from the little that I see with other people. Sometimes the little that a man will just throw aside, the woman may see it in a different way and act up. We don't know whether it's their makeup that makes them so petty... *(Rev Dua)*

While it is true that African women especially view their intimate and marital relationships as very important, and because broken relationships trigger emotional distress in many women (as indicated in the responses of a number of the women survivors in the previous chapter), perceptions of women's gullibility, biological and emotional weakness could lead to attributing emotional or mental distress to the woman victim. The perceived inherent female weakness expressed by the EGP respondents may be either interpreted as proof of women's irresponsibility in their relationships and choice of partners or considered a penchant for ignoring good advice by using their 'hearts' and not their 'heads. I interpret this to mean that women are sometimes seen as abandoning the use of their common sense or intelligence. Compared to men, women are largely perceived as irrational and even petty since '...they are not able to cope with things men see as simple and overlook...'. While this perception may be true for some specific cases, it could also simply be a stereotypical representation of women generally. Further, it may also affect the chosen approach or process of support or treatment. Indeed, this perception may even result in medical help-givers and others such as pastors over-pathologising women's distress.

This is a general concern raised by Richard McNally with respect to mental disorders in the West.[10] In examining women's responses to this perception of EGPs, the shared experiences of the women survivors I interviewed demonstrate that they were no weaklings; neither were they petty or as gullible as perceived. Rather, they came across as women of strength and perseverance, even in affliction. I do not by any means deny individual or general gender differences in physical strength. Concerning emotional strength and intellectual capabilities, however, I am aware of no convincing empirical data that proves mental inferiority or inherent weakness in women.

More importantly, the data suggests that the EGPs appeared not to have applied different approaches in their response to cases of emotional/mental ill-health *on the basis of sex or gender notions*. In effect, their perceptions of women made no difference to their general response to the cases they encountered.

v. Perceived Causes of Emotional/Mental Distress and Illness

The African Christian's strong tendency to uncover the causes of ill-fortune or disease is critical to understand why Christian pastors and congregants would search diligently for the causes of mental health challenges. This theme is identified both from the perspective of the EGP respondents of what causes mental illness and others' comments on causes. To explain the major theme, I have employed the sub-themes of spiritual, physical/biomedical, socio-cultural and multiple or complex causes. Also, under the sub-themes, further categories and themes emerged, depicting the nuances in perceived as well as gender specific causes.

i. Spiritual causes

The perception that mental illness or emotional distress has spiritual causes or undertones, or, at the very least, a spiritual connection seems to be consistent with the African Christian primal religious worldview on misfortunes and diseases. While 8 (40%) of the EGPs referred directly to spiritual causation, all but one of them (95%) spoke about a spiritual factor or connection to mental illness, and narrated some of the cases witnessed or handled. Most of the women survivors (80%) also perceived a spiritual connection to their condition. Other causes cited by the EGP respondents to explain emotional/mental distress and illness include marital problems, poverty, hereditary factors and drug abuse. Spiritual causality or connection was nonetheless a major factor for them. Spiritual causes were mentioned in two categories: (a) those that result from demonic activity, occult or witchcraft attacks, curses and breaking taboos, and (b) those that stem from not having a relationship with God, a weak faith, sin or disobedience. The four (20%) EGPs' views below serve to illustrate category (a):

> So when I get to know that this person who is having a mental problem did something occultic, then I know it is a spiritual problem...
> *(Rev Awuni)*

> Some of our women are barren and they go to juju-men to give them a child. When the child is born, you see that they don't behave normally... *(Rev Dua)*

> Some societies, they have to take you through cultural practice before you reach a certain stage. The person says I am a Christian and refuses to do it and they force the person and something else happens.
> *(Rev Naaba)*

With spiritual problems it can sometimes be a spell cast on somebody...
sometimes the person did something like stealing or something of that
sort, and they are placed under a curse. *(Rev Atta)*

Theresa Wiafe-Asante, who is involved in Christian deliverance ministry
agreed with the views shared above. She was firmly of the opinion that the
devil is behind most distresses and may use the 'thin line between the mental
and spiritual world' to 'push someone in with the intent to destroy them.'[11]
She also recounted how sometimes women accused of witchcraft come to her
to check whether the accusation is true, suggesting that some women may
consider themselves carriers of malevolent spiritual agency, and this thinking
produces grave distress.[12] She was emphatic, though, that not all psychological
illnesses are directly instigated by demonic agents or require deliverance as a
response. It is quite significant that in sharing their theological perspectives
on emotional distress and mental illness, only one of the EGPs (5%) stated
that not all such conditions were caused by demons:

> I believe as a pastor that not all mental illness is demonic so they have
> to also seek mental treatment and support them emotionally.
> *(Rev Ntow)*

That only one out of the twenty EGPs was emphatic about this points
to the persisting, strong belief of the African Christian in the role of malevolent
spiritual forces in ill-fortune and illnesses that are difficult to explain.[13] This
perception may also have led to the conclusion that scholars like Esther
Acolatse have drawn, that African pastors tend to over-spiritualise problems,
particularly emotional distress, hence her insistence on the need to look at
other tools that would both respond to the African Christian's search for
meaning in time of distress and bring the desired relief.[14]

In category (b), the EGPs attributed emotional/mental distress or
illness to spiritual failure, such as weakness, sin or disobedience on the part
of the sufferer:

> In my opinion, one is lack of knowledge; two is lack of spiritual
> empowerment. You can't say you have spiritual empowerment if you
> don't know God... *(Rev Anan)*

> Mental illness/distress may signify unforgiveness. In actual fact, God
> gave us guidelines as to how we should be when it pertains to offenses
> of Christian to Christian... *(Rev Nanor)*

I think they...these things come about as result of sin, people not putting up the right attitude in life and wanting to go wayward, and against the laws of God... *(Rev Onua)*

In fact, one EGP was convinced that a born-again believer cannot suffer mental distress:

If you don't accept Jesus as your Saviour, you will be harassed by the devil based on that. You are under the devil because you have not submitted to the Lordship of Christ. But if you are born again believer, then you will not have this distress, which is a force from the kingdom of darkness... *(Rev Suni)*

Matthew S. Stanford and Kandace R. McAlister show in their work that such perceptions are not limited to African Christians, but also pertain in the Western Church, especially among conservative/evangelical congregations.[15] While personal sin and other related factors in mental illness should not be overlooked, Matthew S. Stanford,[16] Robert H. Albers and his co-authors,[17] Marcia Webb[18] and many other scholars call for a more informed and compassionate view. They recognise the complexity of causes and the need to minister holistically to the afflicted, instead of indicting them.

ii. Physical/biomedical causes

Although the EGPs stressed spiritual causality, seven (35%) of them also perceived mental distress and illness as resulting from physical/bio-medical factors. These include neurological, physiological, hereditary, addictive and unmanaged stress factors, as well as effects of physical illness. Some cited women's biological make-up as a contributory cause of women's mental distress. A few of their views are captured below:

It was then I wanted to know and I found when she was born, she fell and it was biological... *(Rev Awuni)*

Being addicted to drugs like 'wee' and cocaine smoking can also cause it... *(Rev Akyia)*

...[w]e know some people can have those traces from the family lines... *(Rev Atta)*

Sometimes managing stress or challenges can trigger such behaviour if it is not done well. *(Rev Mawu)*

It is interesting that some EGPs also associated children born with mental challenges with their mother's mental frame at the time of pregnancy or their attempts to abort the babies:

It could happen that the woman is pregnant and the one who impregnated her is irresponsible, so the woman will decide to abort it. She attempted it one or two times but the abortion is not successful, this will affect the child biologically when it is born. *(Rev Nsiah)*

...[i]t can be infection in the womb as you see sometimes women are not happy with the pregnancy and try to abort it. Even if they give birth to that child, because they are not happy with the pregnancy the joy in the mother will not come; always bitterness coming through the breast to the child. So right from infancy, you see that child starts having side effects from the mother. *(Rev Atta)*

The phenomenon described above the effects of unsuccessful abortion on babies may be worth investigating, as it appears to be a perception held by many in the Ghanaian community. It is also one which I have heard several times from ordinary persons, pastors and even nurses. Under the same sub-theme, some EGPs linked women's biological make-up to their mental ill-health:

Sometimes their menstrual cycle shifts forward or backwards and this can cause them to be thinking or get worried. Also pains during the menstrual period can also affect their lifestyles and mental stability. *(Rev Doku)*

...[s]ometimes their menstrual period and the issue of menopause... *(Rev Ntow)*

For one EGP verbal abuse from a spouse when a woman is in the process of delivering a baby may trigger mental anguish in her:

...[w]hen about to go through menses, when they get pregnant too; when they are about to deliver and you insult them, that is, the husbands... *(Rev Suni)*

Findings from the research of Vivien K. Burt and Victoria C. Hendrick affirm many of these views.[17]

iii. Socio-cultural causes

Apart from spiritual and physical causes, some respondents equally attributed emotional/mental distress and illness to socio-cultural factors. Social and cultural factors that affect both men and women as well as women-specific factors were cited under this sub-theme. Unfulfilled expectations, poverty, unemployment, lack of education, loss of health and societal demands featured among the issues mentioned. According to the EGPs, marriage and relationship problems appeared to transcend all other such factors for women. They also identified traditions and customs that affected women's mental health. Some of the views on factors that pertained to both women and men are outlined below:

...[s]ometimes poverty and unfulfilled expectations mostly...
(Rev Bia)

There are people who are mentally disturbed due to poverty; some can even be inferiority complex and probably constant harassment ...
(Rev Nanor)

Some marriage problems, stress, joblessness, family issues and sometimes also relationship problem between a parent and a child...
(Rev Doku)

In addition, the EGPs cited inferiority complex arising from lack of education or lack of a life partner as a possible contributor to emotional distress:

Another area is formal education. If the person is not educated and you always bring things that will require an educated response in the congregation, the person will feel ostracised as if she has no value.
(Rev Atta)

...[y]ou know you are growing and no man is coming for you and the pressure [is] coming from society. Seeing your peers marrying, especially in the Christian circle where somebody seems to be keeping to the terms of righteousness, yet nobody proposes; yet those who are flirting about are marrying; it's frustrating... *(Rev Anan)*

Sixteen (80%) of the EGPs mentioned distress stemming from broken relationships during courtship or marriage as another factor. They had so much to say from their pastoral experiences about the negative effects of infidelity, maltreatment and unrealised expectations in such romantic relationships specifically on women's psychological wellbeing. One shared his relative's sad experience:

> This aunt got married to a chief, *Omanhene*. And at a point in time, the chief decided he was not interested in the marriage again. She went completely mad. She was taken to Ankaful Hospital and a lot of places, but she couldn't recover and she eventually died. *(Rev Quao)*

In fact, their husbands' infidelity and a sense of betrayal pushed some of the women the EGPs had ministered to into despair:

> She had married this man for about seven years and they [didn't have] any issues out of the marriage. They were both Christians and were attending the same church. Then outside pressure, family pressure mounting and eventually the young man pulled out and even left the church. He went for another lady, had a child with that lady and this woman had to leave the house. At the time I met the pair, she told me it had gotten to the stage she wanted to commit suicide. *(Rev Osei)*

> I realised that her case had to do with her husband breaking up with her and they have children. She suspected her husband had picked up another woman. *(Rev Awuni)*

> It was a disappointment from a man. They had children but there was neglect from the man. And it appears the woman was giving much love but the response was not coming and there was a sort of total neglect... later on, the man went in for another woman... *(Rev Nanor)*

Another cause of women's distress that was identified was the abuse and maltreatment by their husbands:

> When you consider the way and manner some of the husbands treat their wives, it is so horrible and I think that is what makes them go through those kind [of] distresses... *(Rev Quao)*

> ...[f]rom my ethnic group, no man sees a wife as a partner but a doormat...in sex etc., or else she is beaten for not submitting. Women are beaten into submission. My mother lost all her teeth as a result of this view. I even developed hatred for my father. I saw more abuses of my mother for refusal of sex... *(Rev Suni)*

One EGP cited a broken courtship that had affected a member of his congregation:

> My discussion with her and her family was that a pastor agreed to marry her but it didn't work out and that was how the challenge began. *(Rev Anan)*

The EGPs also mentioned the inimical effects of cultural practices, traditions, norms and perceptions on women. Multiple roles, having no say at both family and public levels were other contributory factors. Also, witchcraft accusation and even violence resulting from such norms and practices were seen to precipitate mental ill-health. Some EGPs were concerned about the implicit acceptance of such gendered patterns of behaviour and practices as part of Ghanaian culture. Below are some of their observations:

> Culturally, men have more sexual freedoms than women and this can have some psychological effects on the woman... *(Rev Doku)*

> In our area here, they force the women into early marriages. This running away to the south is another contributing factor. They run away to become head porters which can cause some of these things... *(Rev Bona)*

> There was a scenario relating to a man dying and leaving the wife. People treat her like she is the cause and that puts emotional stress on the woman. *(Rev Tuuli)*

> We can talk of widowhood rites in marriage and those are main issues that are cultural and very disturbing. *(Rev Prah)*

The EGPs appeared to recognise that the objectification, disrespect, restriction and perception of women as inferior to men were not only manifestations of patriarchy, but had negative emotional and mental impact on women as well. The following cultural perceptions are commonly demonstrated in Ghanaian culture:

> In most instances, the patriarchal society shows the woman as inferior to the man. In that sense, the women have issues that they cannot talk about and are always at the receiving end. *(Rev Ntow)*

> Culturally, some women are seen as witches, people may point fingers at them. Sometimes, too, women are seen as second-class citizens and pushed to the background, not at the forefront of family and national affairs. *(Rev Onua)*

They are restricted; in the house they are seen as [having to] obey their husbands. They do the chunk of the work, even if she is working, she has to do her chores after she returns from work. Then, also, she is always doing what the man says because the man is the boss.
(Rev Awuni)

Culturally, women are downgraded; they are not respected. Even when you go for funerals, women are not supposed to greet, that is their cultural set up; only the men are allowed to talk. In the home, if the man is taking a decision, he doesn't consider what the woman says, what the men say is final, whether the woman agrees to it or not.
(Rev Nsiah)

The socio-cultural factors, including those affecting women in particular, are reflected in several literary sources. Peter Beresford, for one, has stressed the need to consider social factors as highly significant in policy formulation and decision-making that seek to address mental health in Western countries, and not just to depend on the medical approach.[20] This is good advice for African governments as well. The study by Esther D. Rothblum and Ellen Cole places a similar emphasis and raises questions on several socio-cultural dimensions of women's mental health in Africa.[21] In effect, the above factors outlined by the EGP respondents must be considered in conjunction with any attempts to improve mental health states, whether in unemployment, poverty, gender inequality, lack of decision-making power, violence or harmful cultural traditions.

iv. Multiple or complex causes
Two (10%) of the EGPs recognised that emotional distress and mental illness may have complex causes. According to one of them,

> It could be biological, inherited from the family that has it. Spiritual things like demons can also cause a mental problem. If the person is over-stressed or thinks a lot or is worried, it could also affect them psychologically. Social, spiritual economic, material and other issues can also cause it. *(Rev Nsiah)*

In the other's view, the causes go from complex to baffling or mysterious:

> This is a bit complex; but to my understanding, some are caused by we ourselves. Others come by (sic) through coincidence or a spiritual incident. The deliverances I have been in, when you interview people,

some are not of themselves and it happens to them... *(Rev Bona)*

In spite of the multiplicity of factors cited by most of the EGPs as causes of emotional distress and mental illness, their perceptions of causality tend to largely reinforce these factors as products of the religious and cultural context and an African primal imagination that is very much alive, regardless of their exposure to Western religion, education or science. Their recognition of economic and socio-cultural pressures in their daily encounters as possible precipitators of emotional and mental distress also demonstrates their practical engagement with the real issues affecting those to whom they minister. There is an apparent willingness to balance and include helpful perspectives from other contexts in their practice and response.

Summary and Conclusion

The data analysed above presents insights into experiences, perceptions and perspectives which the EGPs, including those training for ministry, generally have about various aspects of emotional and mental distress and illness. These experiences, views and beliefs regarding causality, gender differences and observable symptoms appear to derive from the personal ministry experiences, training, socialisation, as well as cultural and religious context of the EGPs. Many of the pastors I interviewed held similar views. There are however also interesting points of divergence, although not as many as the similarities. In the next Chapter, I continue to explore and analyse other themes that emerged from the data from the interviews with the EGPs. I also examine how they responded to mental health and women's mental health cases, their cultural and theological understanding and perspectives on collaborating with other caregivers, particularly professional MHPs.

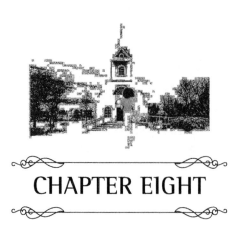

CHAPTER EIGHT

PASTORS RESPONDING: INTERVENTIONS, KNOWLEDGE, COLLABOARATION, THEOLOGICAL AND CULTURAL UNDERSTANDING

Introduction

In this chapter, I analyse the seven remaining themes from my interviews with the EGPs. These are: i) pastoral responses (practical interventions) to address cases of emotional distress/mental illness; ii) the knowledge base of abnormal psychology/mental illness; and iii) cultural perceptions and understanding of emotional distress and mental illness. The rest of the themes are iv) theological perspectives on mental health and distress; v) pastors' and evangelical churches' (E-churches) support for women's roles and for women in distress; vi) perspectives on how evangelical Ghanaian churches must respond; and vii) perspectives on formal collaboration with professional MHPs.

Pastoral Responses (or Practical Interventions) to Address Cases of Emotional/Mental Distress and Illness

This theme comprises the range of responses and practical interventions the EGPs applied in dealing with the mental health challenges of the sufferers they encountered. Spiritual responses were predominant in the practice of the EGPs. It was however obvious that they engaged in other practical interventions to help sufferers. The following sub-themes were used to explain the major theme: Direct medical response, Spiritual responses and Social responses/ interventions. Under the sub-themes identified (except the direct medical response sub-theme), there are further categorisations.

a. Medical Response (Referral) Only

Only one (5%) of the 20 respondents appeared to have made a direct referral to a medical facility without a *prior* intervening spiritual response (such as prayer):

> All things told me something was off and I need[ed] help from a medical officer. So we contacted the medical personnel and they came in to look at him and said they had to take him over there but he did not want to go. He had to be carried out of church to the hospital... *(Rev Dua)*

However, being a pastor, there is every possibility that Respondent 20, Rev Dua, may have also prayed for God's intervention, as this appears to be the practice of most of the EGPs as recounted in their responses. Two such are recorded below:

> My principle is, 'Prayer, number one'. Because we know that God can fix all these things. But when we know that this is more physical, we let the right people handle it. *(Rev Poku)*

> From where I stand as a Pentecostal pastor, we say that every disease has a spirit behind it. So almost any case that comes, ranging from malaria to mental illness or anything that it may be, the first thing we do is to pray and ask God to intervene. Nevertheless, we do know that it is not everything that is spiritual but the first thing is always to pray and then deal with the case... *(Rev Awuni)*

Thus, apart from the one case of direct referral to a medical facility, it is not improbable that the EGPs used prayer together with other spiritual responses catalogued below, to mediate the effects of mental illness/emotional distress.

b. Spiritual Responses

The categories under Spiritual responses are a) Pastoral counselling (with or without prayer); b) Prayer alone; c) Deliverance (casting out demons while also incorporating prayer); d) Multiple spiritual responses (pastoral counselling, prayer and deliverance); (e) Multiple spiritual responses plus referrals to medical/psychological facilities; (f) Whipping and similar practices as part of a spiritual response.

i. Pastoral counselling (with or without prayer):

Eight EGPs (40%) specifically mentioned counselling the sufferers who consulted them. Others used terms such as 'talking' to describe part of their interventions:

> When they brought her to me, we went through some counselling and she calmed down. So she was sober enough to answer my questions. *(Rev Atta)*

> The first day, she didn't talk; it was the second day that she voiced it out. It was a marital problem. As part of the counselling process, I allowed her to talk. *(Rev Ntow)*

> We had to do a lot of talking rather than praying because she needed to hear words of encouragement... *(Rev Osei)*

Counselling as a process of help is a learned skill. Some writers have questioned the adequacy of the pastoral knowledge on counselling in Africa to respond to crises such as emotional/ mental illness or distress. Esther Acolatse, for example, believes that 'formal pastoral training which equips the pastoral counselor to effectively integrate theology and other human and social sciences is too often lacking...'[1] Thus, although a significant number of EGPs mentioned counselling the sufferers, I also question the effectiveness of the process of 'talking' between the EGPs and the sufferers or their families as counselling. Abraham A. Berinyuu, likening the African pastor to a 'diviner',[2] proposes a 'desirable African approach' in which the 'eliciting of information by the healer is itself part of the healing process especially when it is carried out empathetically.'[3] Berinyuu does not however do away with the need to know *how to* counsel. He rather proposes a contextually relevant approach. Obviously, how pastors counsel is another area that needs serious exploratory study, because presumptions of what counselling is could be dangerous, especially for sufferers.[4]

ii. Prayer alone

Four (20%) of the EGPs stated that their only response to a case of emotional/mental distress was prayer. That was brought to their notice. Rev Dua, Respondent 20 related a case of distress which manifested as severe restlessness in a congregant:

> After I prayed with her, and she was settled down, [that] I used Scriptures and prayed over her life...

Respondent 1, Rev Nanor, said he did not have to take a sufferer through deliverance; prayer was enough:

> I prayed for the young man's situation. Sometimes when you know the cause, you hardly call it deliverance.

The strong emphasis on prayer, an indispensable intervention tool for pastors, indicates a firm belief in God's power and willingness to heal all manner of diseases, including emotional/mental distress or illness. It also reflects the worldview of African EGPs, which postulates that the human body, soul and spirit are not compartmentalised. In other words, physical manifestations of disease have spiritual connotations that should be tackled primarily with spiritual responses before or alongside anything else. Christian counsellors and sufferers have confirmed the central role of prayer in a sufferer's life and quest for healing. They however advise against any inappropriate use of prayer in terms of its content and timing, so that pastoral caregivers do not become like 'Job's comforters', using words of condemnation or judgment in the process of prayer.[5] This would apply especially to conditions with symptoms of irrational guilt, shame, worthlessness and obsessions with religious content.[6] An effective application of the principle would therefore require knowledge, good assessment and discernment.

iii. Deliverance (casting out demons while incorporating prayer)

Churches tend to considerably use deliverance or the exorcism of demons in response to emotional distress/mental illness cases, even though it is not done arbitrarily. The EGP respondents described a need-assessment process for this practice. It is however noteworthy that some EGPs asked for help from other more experienced pastors or deliverance practitioners for the ritual to be successfully conducted. In my interviews, eight (40%) of the EGPs specifically mentioned the use of the deliverance ritual in their interventions. Respondent 12 explained why:

> As a pastor, we tend to pray for people, we try to do exorcism because it is biblically okay. Jesus had been exorcising demons from mentally ill people, so usually that is our first approach... *(Rev Poku)*

Other EGPs gave graphic descriptions of some of the cases of apparent mental illness and the positive results obtained from the application of the ritual:

> She was totally insane. She was brought in completely naked and we took this lady through, and [after] prayers and on the third day, by the grace of God, the girl was completely delivered...We were told that

she had been sent to the hospital and [was] taking a lot of drugs, but there was no response. But by the grace of God, we prayed with her just two days and she regained her mind. *(Rev Quao)*

We went for a crusade and the fellow was in chains, and it was through prayer intervention that he came back to life. We were a group who prayed for him. *(Rev Bona)*

One EGP mentioned the belief in the potency of the use of the 'Name of Jesus' in the process of deliverance and stated that he had employed the ritual on the telephone to restore normalcy to a mentally distressed woman:

After establishing the cause, I asked her to put the phone on loudspeaker so that the husband will hear the words I was using to pray and know that I was only using the Name of Jesus and nothing else. The moment I said, 'In the Name of Jesus, I command you spirit of infirmity to leave this daughter of God!', she manifested, and fell [down]. She vomited until everything disappeared and the problem was solved at that point... She is now sober and normal. *(Rev Naaba)*

The EGPs apparently either worked in a team for deliverance or called in help from those who were considered to have a 'calling' to the deliverance ministry. This was the case for two EGPs:

We had a pastors' all-night programme at the church when they brought the case. We prayed but we didn't get results that day. I remember[ed] one young pastor who said he was excellent in deliverance, so I asked him to handle it. He lost his voice and was tired and couldn't. ...So the next Sunday, they brought her to the church service. A colleague of mine helped me and we handled it. We prayed till 8pm before we left the church. She became all right and we took her home... *(Rev Awuni)*

After a short interview, I was able to establish what was happening to her and I called two other prayer members from my church to try a deliverance session. For about three months now, she has been doing very well, by God's grace... *(Rev Naaba)*

The stories from the EGPs' deliverance sessions raise questions of differentiation. Esther Acolatse, a critic of this pastoral practice, faults their tendency to over-spiritualise emotional problems. She observes that 'The strong sense of belief in the unity among the physical, psychical and spiritual is so pervasive that in pastoral situations it is often difficult for the troubled person as well as the healer to see the differentiation that might allow them make a clearer and more accurate diagnosis.[7] While Acolatse affirms that deliverance is legitimate and often effective in freeing people from demonic activity, her emphasis is rather on ministry practitioners developing a more 'robust understanding of the human person that encompasses medical, psychological and spiritual needs, which in turn means developing more finely-tuned tools for pastoral diagnosis.'[8] In the absence of such tools, it is clear from the data that some of these deliverance sessions do produce positive results. Nevertheless, there also are heart-breaking stories of persons, including some of the women respondents I interviewed, who attend deliverance session after session without experiencing any change in their condition. This left them in more perplexity about their faith or salvation.[9]

Still, the serious question of being able to differentiate between spiritually-caused ill-health states and those caused by physical/bio-medical/ psychological factors demands a response. This is because it is the key to positive mental health, especially women's mental health, and equips pastors as first-line responders in the use of careful approaches that help rather than harm the sufferers. A 'one-size fits all' spiritual approach is therefore problematic. For instance, Harold Koenig asserts that '[N]o systematic research shows that exorcism is a successful treatment for patients with schizophrenia or any other severe and persistent mental illness.'[10] While some African pastors may have an issue with this assertion because of the prevailing worldview, Theresa Wiafe-Asante was categorical in our interview that sometimes 'emotional issues look like spiritual issues', affirming the importance of the need to differentiate.[11]

In a further categorisation of this sub-theme, the EGPs spoke quite extensively about how they differentiate between causes and how their responses depend on their assessment of causality. Some EGPs also examined the physiological manifestations in the sufferers they encountered:

> In most cases too, the spiritual ones make the people more violent... In such cases too, it comes and goes. It comes at a particular time and goes. *(Rev Nanor)*

> Some[times] at birth, the child is born mentally distressed and you will know by looking at them. Sometimes it affects their speech and the rolling of the tongues, too. That cannot be spiritual; it is by birth. *(Rev Bia)*

Five EGPs (25%) attributed their discernment for differentiation to the help of the Holy Spirit. Two examples are outlined below:

> We have the Holy Spirit in us as pastors. The pastor is in the Spirit so the Spirit in me is light. It will shine on the person and I can know the kind of spirit that is causing the problem in the person, I will know it directly, unless God doesn't reveal it to me. Otherwise, I can even mention its name or the source of that spiritual effect. *(Rev Atta)*

> Sometimes the person sits in front of you and you will know just by one question that the Holy Spirit drops on your mind. *(Rev Poku)*

One EGP admitted that even though the Holy Spirit helps when the 'matter is spiritual', one may still need training or information to know what to do when the cause is other than spiritual:

> As I said, it is a little difficult because some of the things that are not spiritual may still manifest as spiritual. One thing we rely on fully to take us deep into that is the Holy Spirit. When it is revealed to you, then you know that this matter is spiritual. But if it is not revealed, then as a pastor, if you have training or information from professionals, then you begin to monitor the person carefully to see the sign that will tell you if you need to call doctors. *(Rev Dua)*

It is apparent from the data that many of the EGPs used questions and counselling in the initial stages of their responses in order to differentiate. A few samples illustrate their method:

> I will first question how it happened and what the person had been doing prior to the arising of the problem. So if his life in general has nothing to do with allowing the enemy to infiltrate or the person has nothing he or she harbours within her, and the issues just arises by itself... *(Rev Nanor)*

> I do counselling and interviewing in trying to find out some background checks and if possible linkages with demonic activities and situations where people can go and contact fetish or some other *juju* person... *(Rev Akyia)*

> You can find out from interacting with the person. You can ask certain questions. Sometimes people are quick to tie everything to the spiritual, but it could be something different... *(Rev Osei)*

For some EGPs, differentiating was easy. For others (two of them) who admitted that it was not so easy, they also relied on medical assessment to help them decide the cause of the problem and how to handle it:

> This is very difficult to differentiate, so in most instances, I approach it from the spiritual point of view and also seek for medical attention. *(Rev Ntow)*

> The first attempt is to take the person to the hospital for the doctor to examine him/her mentally. If it is proven that the person is sound, then we take the spiritual aspect and counsel the person through the Word of God and pray with the person. *(Rev Nsiah)*

Some EGPs indicated that they usually would look out for recurring dreams or other non-physical phenomena as Rev Prah stated in the extract below:

> You can only differentiate depending on the case that is before you. If somebody comes to you and says that I go through this experience in my dreams all the time, or I had a problem with this person and this person cast a spell on me, then you could look at it from a spiritual point of view.

For persons who are sceptical about matters of faith, the scientific basis of most of the approaches mentioned above could be adjudged questionable, except perhaps in instances where the question-and-answer method is used with the counselling approach to arrive at causality. However, questions of faith do not amend themselves to science and observable data. The Church has used spiritual gifts and discernment for centuries, and the Scriptures describe the Holy Spirit as the Spirit of truth[12] who also gives the gift of spiritual discernment[13] as He wills. While it is a matter of faith, it is nonetheless critical, however, to protect the sufferer and to prevent abuse and deception. This cannot be overemphasised because of the dangers of counterfeit, over-zealousness and possible over-spiritualisation in dealing with issues of mental illness, as these may have negative consequences for sufferers. It is therefore of utmost importance that EGPs take these realities and the attendant dangers into consideration by ensuring a careful assessment and the use of all appropriate responses as known and applied by them, including spiritual, to address such issues.

iv. Multiple spiritual responses (counselling, prayer and deliverance)
In some of the cases they encountered, the respondents applied a multiplicity of spiritual responses, as in the following example:

> I will first pray and counsel the person. After counselling, then deliverance and prayer, and then I will continue with the counselling through the Word of God. *(Rev Doku)*

> When they brought her to me, we went through some counselling and she calmed down... I called two other prayer members from my church to try a deliverance session. For about three months now, she has been doing very well, by God's grace. *(Rev Naaba)*

v. Multiple spiritual responses and referral to medical/psychological facilities
Significantly, 10 (50%) EGP respondents appeared to apply a multi-pronged approach to address cases of emotional distress/mental illness, which in specific cases included referrals to medical or mental health practitioners:

> In the church, generally, we have mental health workers, even some of the pastors' wives are mental health workers. If the case needs drugs, we hand it over to them to send the person to the hospital aside our prayers. We also follow up with other assistance that will help the person recover...*(Rev Atta)*

> What we do first is the prayer, then deliverance... After prayer when we find out the cause of the problem, [then] we will help the person to seek medical attention. *(Rev Awuni)*

> First, we counselled her and we called the family members to know [her] history. They informed us and we also asked her to go the hospital to check if there is a medical issue. After[wards], we also prayed for her. Now, by the grace of God, she is okay. *(Rev Nsiah)*

When asked their reasons for referring such cases to medical or psychological practitioners in addition to applying pastoral responses, the EGPs were almost unanimous in their assertion that it was not contrary to the Bible to seek medical help. Respondent 2, Rev Mawu emphatically stated:

> I believe that God wants us to be first and foremost informed about what it is all about; then we can refer or prescribe the appropriate remedy. Jesus said that [the] sick has to go to the physician, so he didn't discount the point of physicians being available. God has gifted them

to do that, but still he prayed for people to get healed; so it's both.

The EGPs also acknowledged their limitations as pastors conceded that medical and other professionals have a contribution to make in the healing process, since not all cases have spiritual causes:

> Yes, because I am not a professional. That is why I have been referring people to professionals. What it is not within my means, I will not force myself; I direct the person to the appropriate quarters... *(Rev Quao)*

> ...[b]ecause if it comes to [the] physical like prescribing drugs, I can't do it. Mine is only the prayer and advice that I will offer. If it needs drugs, we refer them to those who are in that department... *(Rev Nsiah)*

Rev Mawu maintained that even if mental illness was caused by factors other than spiritual, both Christian pastors and medical/psychological professionals have specific roles to play to bring about recovery:

> I didn't have any experience because it was the first time... Fortunately, I had one pharmacist, so I decided if I deal with the spiritual aspect, then the pharmacist will also handle any medical issue that may crop up.

The multi-pronged response, as the EGPs outlined in the examples they cited, has important implications for dealing with emotional and mental illness or distress. Evidently, some EGPs were not averse to applying a combination of social, spiritual and medical/psychological responses holistically to address mental distress. Interestingly, the data from the 10 women respondents indicates that 8 (80%) of them were not advised by any of the EGPs they consulted to seek medical or psychological treatment. Yet, in my analysis of the answers of EGP respondents, as we have seen here, a significant number claimed to work actively with professional practitioners in their response to emotional and mental distress.

vi. Use of whipping and similar practices as part of the spiritual response of deliverance

All (100%) the EGP respondents took strong exception to the use of whipping, caning, chaining to trees and other similar practices carried out in some prayer camps and *sunsum sɔre* as part of prescribed spiritual exercises in responding to sufferers. The EGPs were unequivocal about the unscriptural nature of these practices as the following extracts show:

It is not biblical and once Jesus didn't practise it, I feel it should not be encouraged. Jesus said, 'Go and cast it out'; he didn't say, 'Go and whip them'. *(Rev Bona)*

Jesus met a madman who broke his chains. It was the people who chained him, not Jesus. *(Rev Atta)*

Others believed that the practices were an abuse of the human rights of sufferers and would therefore require the intervention of the State:

...[y]ou are just punishing the person's body and I think such people should be arrested... *(Rev Awuni)*

[T]he fact that a person is mentally ill or challenged does not mean that they don't have human rights. *(Rev Osei)*

Two (10%) EGPs felt the practices were senseless:
It is a spiritual issue, so if you are beating the patient or the sick person, you are hurting his or her body, it doesn't affect the spirit... *(Rev Bia)*

That is even more demonic than what is happening to the person. If it is a spiritual thing, how can we use the physical to treat it? It doesn't work... *(Rev Dua)*

The accounts of the women survivors underscore the seriousness of such treatment and how it further denigrates sufferers who already have to deal with the indignities of illness and societal stigma. The data seems to suggest, though, that evangelical Ghanaian pastors do not subscribe to such practices, as they did not emerge during the women respondents' engagement with the EGPs either. Thus, it may not be fair to conclude that the EGPs I interviewed, generally speaking, are guilty of such practices. It also appears from the women's data that prayer centres led by persons of evangelical persuasion are not associated with such practices, but this needs further investigation. With the Human Rights Watch Report[14] pointing to the existence of these practices in some churches and prayer camps, I believe the EGPs should join the advocacy to abolish these and other similar practices inimical to mental health of all persons.

c. Social Responses/Interventions

Ten (50%) EGPs reported that they addressed the needs of persons with mental illness/emotional distress by offering different kinds of social support, wherever necessary. This support would usually include financial and material assistance, as well as visits to the sufferers by the church leadership and members. The goal of these actions was to reduce the pain of loneliness and to give the sufferers a sense of belonging and of being loved:

> [S]ometimes there are people who may not be financially sound, so we come in to support. We also encourage the brethren to get close to them and interact to make them feel more at home. And we also support by visiting the house to help in a few things, members are encouraged to do that... *(Rev Akyia)*

> I spoke to the leaders too about it and I spoke to committed and matured people in the church about her, so that we can support her. So that if we even see that she is doing something that is unacceptable by our standards, we should know [that] that is her problem and see how best we can help her. *(Rev Anan)*

> We make sure if they are not in church, we follow up to know why they are not. We make them feel that they belong because loneliness can make them feel abandoned. *(Rev Awuni)*

One EGP appeared to have built a close relationship with a distressed congregant:

> What I did was to invite her to become my friend. I built confidence in her so she could become a friend of mine. She discussed everything with me, and to her, she has no problem. She would not go to hospital for treatment, so I had to convince her and take her to hospital myself and make sure that she is taken care of and bring her back...*(Rev Onua)*

It is clear from the above account that while the actions of this EGP may have resulted from his assessment of the case and projected response, building such a close relationship, especially if the distressed is of the opposite sex, may actually pose the danger of dependency or transference of affection. In fact, it may even result in an inappropriate sexual relationship. As one renowned Christian counsellor and author cautions,

> Whenever two people work closely together on a common goal, feelings of camaraderie and warmth often arise between them. Frequently, these feelings of warmth have a sexual component, including sexual

attraction between counselor and counselee... the wise counselor makes special effort to maintain self-control.[15]

While I am not saying this is what happened in the case of this EGP, pastoral caregivers are often warned about such dangers during the training for counsellors. Indeed, all caregivers need to take this caution seriously to avoid ethical and moral compromises in their interventions.

In all, it is clear that social responses are critical to improve the conditions of mental ill-health. Koenig affirms this function and encourages clergy and churches to make it a part of their ministry.[16] If sensitively offered, such responses also protect sufferers from stigmatisation, especially by church members, particularly if they see their pastors and leaders draw the sufferers close or visit them personally. This re-echoes the Apostle Paul's admonition to 'bear each other's burdens, and so fulfil the law of Christ.'[17] Social responses however come with economic costs in the provision of food and clothing, support to pay hospital fees and so on. This can always be factored into regular church budgets and members could be asked to contribute towards such worthwhile purposes.

EGPs' Knowledge base of Abnormal Psychology/Mental Illness

The importance of the information and data under this major theme derives from the stated premise of this study, that is, to determine whether a lack of understanding and knowledge in pastoral caregivers of mental health and women's mental health issues may actually result in pastoral interventions which perhaps cause more harm than good to sufferers.

Some experts and scholars, emphasise the need for pastors to be well equipped with the knowledge on emotional/mental distress and illness issues.[18] This is not for the purpose of professional diagnosis, but to gain a reasonable understanding of symptoms of distress in order to make appropriate decisions regarding their response.[19]

To assess the EGPs' knowledge base in abnormal psychology or knowledge obtained from a formal educational or training programme on mental illness/emotional distress, I identified three themes which emerged from their responses to the interview questions: a) the pastors' knowledge of any mental disorders; b) their understanding of the nature of 'emotional distress', and 'mental illness'; and c) a self-assessment of their personal capacity to respond to such cases.

The responses showed that the EGPs had very limited knowledge of the formal categories of mental illness/emotional distress, an honest admission they made in their interview answers. Only one (5%) of the twenty EGPs was able to mention one known mental disease. Notwithstanding their inadequate knowledge, they demonstrated a relatively good understanding of what constitutes emotional distress and mental illness in the description of the symptoms. Most of the EGPs were also honest enough to admit they did not have the requisite training to respond appropriately.

a. Knowledge of formal categories of diseases/mental illness

Six (30%) of the interviewed EGPs confessed that they simply did not know or could not name any mental/psychological disease, illness or disorder. Two such responses are captured below:

> Ermm... please pass it on... [laughter] *(Rev Anan)*

> No, I don't know, because if I say something, I will be a liar... *(Rev Bona)*

Some EGPs made an attempt to answer the question by describing symptoms they had observed:

> I have seen quite a number. I have seen the type that is very violent and uncontrollable. I only know the description, not the medical terms for them... *(Rev Naaba)*

> I am not sure but would even probably classify [it as] depression, oppression, suppressions... *(Rev Osei)*

> We can term it madness; that is the general name we call it. *(Rev Atta)*

> Apart from what I will describe as traditional ones, the drug addiction (wee), lack of sleep, loss of inner peace, people who are easily disturbed... *(Rev Prah)*

Still others claimed they could not remember any mental diseases, or that the names were too technical:

> [I]t's technical, so I won't be able to... *(Rev Nsiah)*

> I talk to doctors but I don't know the categorisations. I always ask them what the different types of mental disorder are. They mention those long names and I can't I remember this one or that one. *(Rev Awuni)*

> I may not be able to classify them... *(Rev Poku)*

One EGP tried hard to name one disorder, but did not quite succeed: There is a psychological mental disorder... *(Rev Awuni)*

Thus, only Respondent 6, Rev Akyia, could name one known disorder as classified. He also happened to be the EGP with a doctorate degree:

Schizophrenia is the only one I can remember at the moment.

According to their profiles, the EGPs had received theological training and some mentioned taking courses in Counselling. However, their responses seem to suggest that their curriculum content may have been inadequate in the area of knowledge about mental health. It is possible that as older persons, they may have forgotten what they had been taught. In the short term, refresher training for the EGPs would take care of this apparent inadequacy.

i.   *EGPs' understanding of 'emotional distress'*
In a further exploration of the major theme, all the EGPs described what they understood as 'emotional distress'. Under this theme, I examined the EGPs' understanding of the continuum between minor issues of mental ill-health and more serious cases of mental illness. A range of their responses is given below, starting with those from the EGPs who focused on the sufferer's state of mind:

> ...[w]hen your brain becomes obsessed with unhappy situations. The situation poisons the brain so they become unstable and malfunctioned... *(Rev Atta)*

> ...[h]aving some challenge and not having the ability to share it with anybody and stores it up for a long time. It has a psychological effect on the person and disorganises the person mentally, probably due to mental fatigue. *(Rev Nanor)*

Others centred their understanding on psycho-somatic symptoms of distress:

> When a person's not at ease... he doesn't feel comfortable...*(Rev Bia)*

Some EGPs described 'emotional distress' as the obvious absence of peace or the presence of inner turmoil or pain:

> ...[a] state where you don't have peace and beyond that stage, then you are emotionally traumatised *(Rev Mawu)*

...[t]he person is carrying loads that are weightier than the mind can handle and it is breaking the fellow apart...*(Rev Poku)*

...[t]he fellow is hurt or injured within the inner being. *(Rev Bona)*

...[h]e feels the pain of disappointment, mistrust, betrayal. There is hurt in the inside. *(Rev Tuuli)*

Still others defined the phrase as having to do with unmanaged or uncontrollable situations, excessive worry or stress:

...excessive worry leading to a stage where the person is not even able to think right at the right time. They are not mentally ill, but you realise that sometimes they make funny decisions. *(Rev Osei)*

[W]hen people are in an emotional disturbance, you find them creating some other problems for themselves. Things that don't exist, they treat them as if they exist in their life. *(Rev Dua)*

Two of the respondents described 'emotional distress' as a state of unease, without referring to a probable cause. Others obviously considered the sufferers as contributing to their condition by 'allowing' it:

The person is not thinking right because there is a stress that has come upon him/her. It is because he/she is allowing a misunderstanding of an issue and emotionally [is] being distressed by it. *(Rev Suni)*

...it's a situation where one is not able to control his/her emotions and allow[s] whatever circumstance he (sic) is facing to take the better part of them and therefore [is] unable to, [in quotes] 'think right'. *(Rev Akyia)*

From the theological perspectives shared by the EGPs, the factor of 'allowing' oneself to become emotionally distressed is projected through the belief by more than half of the respondents (55%) that emotional/mental illness happens only to people who are either not spiritually strong or do not have enough faith.

ii. EGPs' understanding of what constitutes 'mental illness'
In their descriptions of 'mental illness', six (30%) of the EGPs understood it as presenting themore serious symptoms of mental ill-health, particularly in

those with psychotic features, as postulated by Koenig in *Faith and Mental Health*.[20] Some of the respondents' explanations are outlined below:

> ...[w]here [a] person is no more himself/herself and that she (sic) can go out naked and begin to talk... *(Rev Anan)*

> ...[t]he person goes beyond the normal. Nothing good seems good to the person. The person behaves in a very awkward way and sometimes can harm, or be sober. *(Rev Naaba)*

> People within that category may be found making or speaking words that you can't put together to make meaning. And sometimes the way they behave, their dressing. Just yesterday when I was driving, I saw a man along the way. I saw a man who passed by and picked something from the floor (sic) and put it straight into his mouth. Automatically, when you see such a person, you know that he is out of his mind. *(Rev Mawu)*

Three EGPs (15%) pointed to the possibility of biological or chemical factors being responsible for the condition:

> The person has a disease of the brain, such as forgetfulness, does not respond to social cues or delays in responding. *(Rev Doku)*

> I can equate it as a disease that causes imbalance. *(Rev Akyia)*

> ...[a] biological disorder. That makes the person mentally unfit to discharge his/her own duties in life. *(Rev Ntow)*

Still, seven respondents (35%) believed that it involves a malfunction of the psyche or reasoning:

> It has to do with abnormality within the mental faculty... *(Rev Awuni)*

> It is when a person can't reason well. He may says *(Rev Bia)*

> ...[w]hen there is a disorder in the mind-set of a person, that the person has a mind-set that is affecting his well-being or proper reasoning. *(Rev Tuuli)*

One EGP (5%) associated it with a lack of understanding or inability to act quickly on a distressing matter:

I will think it has to do with understanding or ill understanding. I will say that lack of understanding of an issue is mentally distressing. It is not because the thing is stressful, but you don't apply the right knowledge to the situation. So, mentally, you are ill. *(Rev Suni)*

The state of mental ill-health actually ranges from what may be viewed as minor emotional disturbances to major psychotic illnesses, according to the classification found in formal diagnostic manuals of psychiatric disorders.[21] Pastoral caregivers like the EGP respondents are often confronted with cases of people who suffer anything from minor neuroses to serious schizophrenia, and they are expected to somehow provide effective solutions. The very fact that pastors attempt to intervene, irrespective of the levels of severity of mental illness, necessitated my exploration of their understanding of the range of such conditions. As the data has shown, they appear to be aware of this continuum, even if not in the formal sense. Under the themes of Pastoral Response and Collaboration, the EGPs were further given the opportunity to explain how they assessed the cases that were brought to them in order to determine the ones that needed more than their pastoral intervention skills and what they did when confronted with such cases.

b. *Perception of the capacity (level of knowledge and skill) to respond*
Twelve (60%) of the EGP respondents said they had either had no training, or whatever they had was inadequate. As two EGPs stated,

> Not sure I have the training...I can say that I don't have formal training, but on the job though gave me that especially... but that is never adequate...*(Rev Nanor)*

> ...[b]ack at the seminary, we had mental doctors come there to give us talks on these issues. We had a few [talks]; I wouldn't say it was an intensive programme, just talks. I don't have enough experience or training ... *(Rev Mawu)*

Only two EGPs (10%) submitted that their theological training had addressed some aspects of psychology:

> What I did was Clinical Counselling and we were open to basic medical procedures. I did it as a different course in addition to my pastoral training. In the theological training, we looked at some aspect of that. I would say, yes. *(Rev Dua)*

When we trained too, we did general counselling and theological counselling... *(Rev Prah)*

The EGPs admitted that they needed training, even where they thought their response was adequate. Below is a sample of their responses:

It is something I wanted to know about because I realise that in my pastoral work, there are people that are attracted to my ministry... I don't have the training. I only have the love. *(Rev Anan)*

I need it [training]; I really need it because we are working with human beings and anything can happen and we will be stranded. So, if you can help us, we will be grateful. This interview has enlightened me on these issues and I have also realised that I don't know much about mental health issues. *(Rev Doku)*

Nine (45%) of the respondents said even though they did not have any training or that it was inadequate, they would know what to do with such cases because they read books. They would also refer the cases to others or depend on the Holy Spirit's help, as some of their extracts suggest:

I have some professionals in church and [I] interact with them. So, at least it has given me some knowledge. *(Rev Akyia)*

All that I have is the experience I got from the senior pastors that I have been using. *(Rev Ntow)*

...[i]f it is beyond spiritual and normal counselling, then I refer to the appropriate profession. *(Rev Osei)*

My simple answer is the help of Holy Spirit. *Rev Bona)*

The EGPs' inability to demonstrate some knowledge of mental illness categories, while claiming that they could recognise it when they saw it, has certain implications. On the one hand, this is positive, because their ability to describe symptoms of emotional/mental distress and illness indicates that they were familiar with some symptoms which manifest when such conditions are present. On the other hand, their inability to identify even basic mental disorders should be of concern, as this may undermine their capacity to determine what could actually be happening in a particular case enough to be able to differentiate between symptoms. They may also ascribe bad or poor behaviour to persons who may actually be distressed or ill and therefore need their support.

Moreover, some of the EGPs' descriptions fit into the typical picture of mental illness, observed on the streets of Ghana and depicted in popular media, of dishevelled and unkempt people, talking 'to the air' unlike the 'nice looking, calm, educated Christian women'. This stereotypical imaging may make it difficult to accept that the latter may also be going through mental struggles. Their ignorance or inadequate knowledge may also undermine the confidence of those who go to them for help. As one woman respondent explained earlier:

> They don't even know what it is. So if you go to a pastor and say, 'I have a bipolar problem', he will say, 'What is that?' And you the mentally ill person has to explain to the pastor. He doesn't have a clue, so how does he advise you? (Rita)

The EGPs' honesty about their lack of expertise or inadequate training is therefore commendable. They acknowledged their need for more education and better training. Indeed, under the current legal regime in Ghana, they would apparently have no option but to be retrained in order to legitimately continue with their counselling interventions.[22] A reading of the relevant law shows that churches would have to be compliant with its provisions and would therefore need to prepare to make such training available to pastors.

EGPs' cultural perceptions and understanding of emotional distress and mental illness

Since Jesus Christ is encountered within our culture, we are saved in it and not out of it. EGPs are Christians and ministers who come from and serve within their Ghanaian and African cultural contexts and consciousness. The main theme explored here, therefore, is the EGPs' cultural perceptions and understanding of emotional distress and mental illness. This theme was categorised into three sub-themes. The first explored the question of prevailing cultural perceptions and concepts about emotional/mental distress and illness in the ethnic background of the EGPs, as well as the treatment given to sufferers in those contexts. The second explored the same question from the context of the EGPs' areas of ministry, while the third sub-theme examined the EGPs' personal cultural convictions and understanding about these issues.

In order to analyse the data under the first two sub-themes, I first extracted the EGPs' perceptions and understanding of their ethnic background as reflected in their views. Then, I proceeded to delineate their views about the treatment of sufferers. I followed the same process in the discussion to determine their perceptions pertaining to their areas of ministry.

a. Understanding from the ethnic background and perceptions

The data suggests a broad similarity of perceptions and understanding of emotional/mental distress and illness. The response to, or treatment of, sufferers also appears to be similar, despite the different ethnic backgrounds of the EGPs. The few notable differences in perceptions and treatment were also recorded. Six EGPs (30%) focused on the spiritual connotations and the way people view such conditions with fear and suspicion, which affects even their family and social relationships:

> ...[s]o, for instance, somebody is even going to marry, they will go and say, 'Do you have mental illness problems in the family?' If [there] is, then it is a no-go area... (Rev Akyia)

> They view it as a spiritual effect. Sometimes it's in the background of the parents. The way they kill people using juju and things like that. Sometimes, if they have killed a madman before in our area, we believe that somebody will be mad in the family. (Rev Atta)

> The... [name of ethnic group deleted] view mental illness as a curse and an abomination that they don't want to accept [it] in the family. When people like that die, they don't mention it because they are bringing some kind of curse into the family. (Rev Poku)

In response to the question, 'How does your ethnic group treat people with mental illness?', the EGPs linked their perceptions of spiritual causality to corresponding forms of treatment or response:

> They do consultation with spiritists to see what the problem is... The person is asked to bring some items for the process. If after three times, nothing happens, the person is abandoned. (Rev Suni)

> Among the... [name of ethnic group deleted], when mental distress happens, the first place is the shrine, to find out the cause of the mental illness and the direction the sorcerer would give. (Rev Nanor)

> They have witch doctors, the *tindan* who are the owners of the land. Where I come from...[name of ethnic group deleted], there are these

people who are said to be specialised in treating mental disorder. The person is sent to any of these places and is left there. This is similar to the prayer camp system. *(Rev Awuni)*

Societal stigma against the sufferer is quite real, according to three EGPs:

...[w]ith that, nobody will mind you or take care of you. And if you misbehave, they will beat you up... *(Rev Atta)*

Culturally, if you are mad, they don't see you as a normal person who can contribute meaningfully. *(Rev Prah)*

There are indicators, however, that not all ethnic groups maltreat the mentally ill, no matter what they consider to be the cause:

They don't drive them away, sometimes if they need food and they approach, they are given. They consider them as part of the community. Some of them may also take the mentally ill people to spiritual churches for prayers. *(Rev Bia)*

...[t]hey accept them and they also help them. Interestingly, they still see them as family members and part of them. So they support them and sometimes, they cook and ask people to give to the person in that situation. *(Rev Osei)*

b.   *Understanding from the area of ministry and perceptions*

The analysis of the EGPs' responses under this sub-theme indicates that a few differences emerged in the areas of ministry. On the whole, however, they simply reflect the perceptions and understanding from the ethnic background. Here also there are a few notable exceptions. In some ministry areas, for instance, the blame was put on the sufferers:

People will always attribute maybe the wrong doings of that person, whether a sin, duped someone or did this or that wrong; that is why he or she is suffering. So they are neglected. *(Rev Mawu)*

They see it as coming from the background or the person has done something wrong or evil and someone cursed him. *(Rev Quao)*

In other areas, the people focused on hereditary traits or ancestral curses:

They will however like to first of all trace if there are any traits of mental illness in the family. If there are traces, they easily conclude that it is a family thing, so they might be under some curse as a family. *(Rev Nanor)*

...some believe that it is a curse from the ancestors and some of them are given to their ancestors. Earlier on, I was told that some were even killed. But in the modern day now, they are not being taken good care of as they should be...*(Rev Anan)*

The EGPs had much to say about how the people from their areas of ministry respond to or treat the mentally distressed. A few of their responses are captured below:

They can be taken to the witchdoctor; some people don't understand and they think they are witches... *(Rev Poku)*

The prayer camp is sought for leaving ill relatives there – it's not really about help. This is not real transformation but religiosity. *(Rev Suni)*

The societal stigma is equally real for sufferers in the EGPs ministry contexts:

In the area that my church is located, they also shy away from you and avoid you... how they give you food to eat, how they treat you, it just will tell you that you are mad. *(Rev Prah)*

When you are not behaving well, you become an outcast in the society, people don't tend to like your company and you are shunned
(Rev Poku)

[s]ome, too, think the mentally ill have been used for rituals and other things. So, you see school children mocking them and elders giving food in dirty things to them. The person is concerned that they should eat, but they don't put it in any hygienic thing because the person is on the floor or at the rubbish dump... *(Rev Tuuli)*

This comment by Rev Tuuli, Respondent 18, is affirmed by the harrowing experience of one of the women respondents in interviewed.[23] However, it is noteworthy that the response and treatment differ in some communities where the EGPs ministered.

In our area, because it is a Muslim community, they try to sympathise with the people.[24] *(Rev Bona)*

In this area, people with mental issues are not harassed or disturbed and they help each other by giving them food and clothing. *(Rev Doku)*

What I have observed they do is they try to consult powerful people, so to speak, that [is], those who have the power to handle them. If it doesn't work, eventually, they report the case to the hospital and the person is sometimes sent to the mental hospital. They don't maltreat the person; I have never seen that. *(Rev Naaba)*

There is no doubt that modernity, education and Christianity have influenced both the cultural perception about and treatment approaches for the emotionally/mentally distressed or ill, even though the religious and cultural worldview still predominates in the ethnic and ministry communities of the respondents. This affirms John Mbiti's observation that Africans will continue to 'resort to both hospitals and medicine-men without a feeling of contradiction.'[25] The EGPs were very aware of these contradictions, as the following interview extracts indicate:

In the past, the reception was not good. But of late, as they have seen a lot of things, when they are taken to the hospital in the early stages, something can be done for them. They try to hide them from the public... *(Rev Dua)*

...[b]ecause of education, Christianity and travelling, the situation is different. That is why we would first of all probe into the causes before resorting to either the shrine, hospital or the church. *(Rev Nanor)*

...now there is enlightenment, so people try to send them to the hospital. The only problem is that they believe that they are outcasts or they believe that they are sick. So after doing it once, twice or thrice, they just leave it there and allow you to just walk about. *(Rev Anan)*

Because the EGPs' responses regarding cultural perceptions appear to feature the usual 'face' of mental illness in Ghana, it is difficult to distil from their responses the prevailing cultural perceptions and treatment of persons who, although not exhibiting all those outward symptoms, may yet be suffering from debilitating conditions such as major depression or anxiety. Many of such persons are mothers and fathers, wives and husbands, caregivers and workers. Further investigation is required to know how to identify such mentally distressed or ill persons and, once identified, how to treat them.

c. *EGPs' personal cultural understanding and perceptions*

The data shows that the EGPs are not only products of their culture, but also products of modern education, Western Christianity and scientific advancement. Even though they largely assented to spiritual causality associated with the cultural perceptions of their ethnic and ministry communities, they differed on the treatment responses, such as the use of sorcerers and traditional shrines. It is interesting that under this theme, a few EGPs disagreed both with seeing the issue as solely spiritual and with seeking only spiritual solutions, even if apparently Christian, such as leaving sick relatives at prayer camps. Their disagreement with the spiritual causality response of people in their ethnic and ministry communities appears somewhat contradictory, judging from their own perceptions of causality. Nonetheless, they were all (100%) against the neglect and maltreatment of sufferers, as well as their stigmatisation. The extracts that follow represent some of the EGPs' responses to the question: 'In what way do you differ from the cultural perceptions and treatment of persons with emotional/mental distress or illness by people from your ethnic background and areas of ministry?'

One EGP totally disagreed with the cultural perceptions emanating from his area of ministry because, according to him, they 'stigmatise' the mentally ill and he would 'want nothing to do with them':

> I don't agree with them on anything. I differ about their approach to those who have mental problems. *(Rev Ntow)*

For Respondent 9, Rev Atta, it was time to shift from the perception that all mental illnesses are spiritually caused:

> They rather resort to spiritual things; meanwhile it may not be a spiritual issue, but biological. I differ on the view because not all mental illnesses are caused by spirits...

Thirteen EGPs (65%) who also said they differed in their perceptions from their communities emphasised the role of the Christian church and pastor in the community as healing resources for the population. They stressed the use of prayer as well as encouraging medical intervention where necessary:

> ...[b]ut first see the doctor, and if there is no solution, then bring it to church, or while the person visits the doctor, the pastor is also informed for prayer to be offered... *(Rev Nanor)*

I will wish that they care for them and take them to the hospital. I also prefer that they can seek for divine intervention by praying at prayer centres but not to be chained or beaten... *(Rev Bia)*

Two of the EGPs (10%), appeared to have no faith in traditional healing resources, presumably sought from shrines:

I just don't agree with the way they see and treat it, because even if it is spiritual the devil cannot cast out demons, it is not possible. So, even if there is that perception of spiritual attack, it should be the name of Jesus that can save that person... *(Rev Awuni)*

Where I want to differ is where the situation arises, they want to tackle it from the traditional side, but hardly do they get any success stories there. Later, they end up sending the person to the hospital... *(Rev Naaba)*

Only one EGP admitted that he shared the some of the same perceptions as his communities. He was however concerned about the marginalisation of survivors of mental illness and distress:

I agree with them to some extent. But they will have to do more because some who recover find it difficult to get any leadership roles or even being asked about their opinions or ideas. *(Rev Dua)*

The EGPs' emphasis on the use of the church's resources alongside those of the hospitals and medical interventions counteracts any attempts by families and communities to seek help from traditional shrines and healers. This is the import of the statement by Rev Awuni above, '...even if it's spiritual, the devil cannot cast out demons...', made in the belief that such traditional resources cannot be of God. This suspicion of traditional healing resources is echoed in the aversion Rev Naaba expressed to receiving help from traditional shrines: '...hardly do they get any success story there.' However, as Berinyuu points out, Christian pastors should be aware that, in a time of grave and inexplicable distress or prolonged illness, their converts may have many questions which stem from their religio-cultural universe, such as the possibility of being bewitched, cursed or forced to pay for ancestral misdeeds. These fears cannot be overlooked or dismissed. Thus, Berinyuu believes that pastors must find ways of responding to such questions from a place of recognition and understanding. They should adopt pastoral care and healing practices that the sufferers can relate to within their context. These practices may also become, he maintains, '*kerygmatic* to the whole community'.[26]

In sum, it is clear from the discussion under this main theme that the African worldview of a spiritual universe that influences perceived abnormal behaviour is widely held and it, in turn, encourages the attitudes, treatment and response towards sufferers. Victim-blaming also appears to be a feature of the cultural perceptions, as well as stigma and abusive treatment in some areas. Nonetheless, there are also good stories of help, support and sympathy.

Theological Perspectives of EGPs on Mental Health and Mental Distress/Illness

The EGPs I interviewed shared their theological reflections and thinking on emotional/mental distress and illness, as well as their use of personal faith and spirituality in addressing such conditions. Accordingly, this main theme is categorised under the following sub-themes and statements: a) mental distress and illness is a result of humankind's original sin/disobedience; b) salvation includes prevention from or healing for mental illness/distress; c) mental illness/distress signifies non-conversion, a reprobate lifestyle or personal disobedience to God; d) the search for/reliance on material possessions may be a factor; e) mental illness/distress does not afflict the spiritually strong or mature; f) mental illness signifies an inability to deal with everyday burdens or worries; g) mental illness/distress can be overcome by persons with strong faith and a close relationship with God; h) faith and spirituality used presumptuously or wrongly can have negative consequences; i) faith and spirituality used in combination with community support and other biblical practices has a positive effect; j) exercising Christian faith and spirituality is not incompatible with seeking medical help; k) not all mental illness is caused by demons; and, finally, l) the mentally distressed are also created by God and must be accepted.

a. *Mental illness or distress is a result of humankind's original sin/disobedience*

Many Christian scholars, theologians and mental health experts[27] agree with the EGPs who believed that emotional/mental distress and illness are the result of humankind's rebellion and brokenness:

> When God created the world, he put all things into it and he wanted us to follow his will. What we see now with the emotional disturbances and sicknesses is because we have gone out of his will to do things on our own. *(Rev Anan)*

God didn't create man with mental disorder but because of sin: illness, diseases and sickness have intruded in human life... *(Rev Atta)*

b. Salvation includes prevention from or healing for mental illness/distress

Rev Atta, Respondent 9, was emphatic that there was a link between one's status of salvation and one's mental health:

> ... God didn't leave man alone, but provided Christ and said anyone who believes in him shall be saved. Being saved doesn't mean just coming to Christ. It means being healed of diseases and illnesses. That is why the Bible says, 'By his stripes, we have been healed'.

c. Mental illness/distress signifies non-conversion, a reprobate lifestyle or personal disobedience to God

Five EGPs (25%) readily linked the presence of mental distress or illness to sin in a person's life:

> ...[e]specially in Romans 12:1-2, we should treat our bodies as living sacrifices to God and change our minds to accept Christ as our personal Saviour, so that people will have peace in their minds. *(Rev Doku)*

> I think they... these things come about as result of sin, people not putting up the right attitude in life and wanting to go wayward and against the laws of God. *(Rev Onua)*

Several writers have challenged this issue of mental illness being a consequence of sin and disobedience in the sufferer's life. Marcia Webb, Matthew S. Stanford and others caution against the further wounding of sufferers through this notion. Without compromising the fact that all humans have sinned and are in need of salvation, Webb is of the view that '...prompted by a particular sort of superficially religious encouragement, these sensitive persons will readily conjure up any number of "sins" for which they might imagine themselves now to be suffering with mental illnesses.'[28]

Stanford agrees with Webb,[29] but also recognises that bad habits and sinful choices could lead to mental challenges, as some EGPs clearly affirmed regarding the use of drugs and alcohol,[30] as well as get-rich-quick schemes:

> ...[i]f you take and abuse drugs, including alcohol and you get some of these things, it is your own doing. You sowed and you are reaping. *(Rev Akyia)*

Then pertaining to those who are craving for money, through that, they became affected because the Bible frowns seriously on those doing 'Sakawa'[31]... *(Rev Nanor)*

d. Search for/reliance on material possessions as a possible factor in the Prosperity Gospel

Unbridled materialism gets people into trouble and affects their mental wellbeing, was the view of five of the EGPs (25%). Of these, one blamed the persons involved, while another blamed the contemporary 'prosperity theology' teaching in some churches:

> Some are rushing to wealth, power, rushing for too many things that we find it difficult to understand. When you hit a wall, that is when these challenges begin to come... *(Rev Naaba)*

> ...[w]hen you think beyond what you are supposed to think of, you get that mental problem... The pastors should preach the full gospel. It shouldn't be one-sided. What we see these days is about money and prosperity... *(Rev Nsiah)*

Even though Wilfred A. Agana[32] and J. Kwabena Asamoah-Gyadu[33] do not necessarily connect emotional/mental distress and illness with the prosperity teaching found mainly among new independent/Charismatic churches, they are however equally concerned that any teaching which focuses primarily on material blessings and prosperity as signs of success in the Christian life or divine approval has negative consequences. These include Christians believing that they cannot be affected by troubles and therefore lacking the tools to deal with troubles and trials when they come, as they are inevitable in life.[34] The inordinate ambition to get wealth certainly would come with anxieties of the kind that Christ warns against in Matthew 6:25-34. If left unchecked, this materialistic mind-set can lead to both physical and mental health problems.

e. Mental illness/distress does not overcome the spiritually strong or mature

Another view which resonated with the EGPs and appeared to be accepted by eleven (55%) of them is that spiritually mature or strong people cannot be overcome by emotional/mental illness:

> What you have on the inside will help you with the stresses from without. So people who have a lot of spiritual energy in them are able

to handle this stress more than those who are quite empty... When you don't have much in you, those things will overcome you... *(Rev Poku)*

I think the more matured you are as a believer, a Christian, you will be able to handle situations. When somebody is matured and knows how to cast his/her burdens upon the Lord, definitely, the manifestation or whatever it is will differ. *(Rev Akyia)*

In any case, the prophets Elijah and Jeremiah could not be described as immature or weak, yet they faced personal emotional struggles. Even Jesus experienced anguish and trouble in His soul.[35] Even if these were not related to any specific illness, they denoted painful emotional experiences. The writer of the Letter to the Hebrews asserts that the Son of God is able to sympathise with all our weaknesses because He went through them, too.[36] Spiritual immaturity is no doubt costly, but spiritual maturity or strength may not necessarily guarantee immunity to grave emotional disturbances. In this respect, therefore, the theology of the EGPs may need to be re-examined in the light of Biblical evidence and from the narratives of the women survivors I interviewed.

f. Mental illness signifies inability to deal with everyday burdens or worries:

Eight EGPs (40%) had much to say about people 'thinking too much' or 'allowing' themselves to be burdened and how this impacts their mental health. Below are typical statements:

The Bible says that we should not be burdened with anything. So if you allow yourself to be burdened, then, of course, you may be having some problems that will lead you somewhere you are not prepared to go... *(Rev Quao)*

...[i]f you think too much, you will have psychological problems. Just leave everything to God. *(Rev Nsiah)*

Again, these assumptions have been challenged. I have personally known cases of mental illness, including my own experience, which did not stem from everyday burdens and worries. These include a sudden onset of mental illness such as anxiety or bipolar disorders, neurological conditions of autism and PTSD due to sexual or other abuse, as well as exposure to extraneous circumstances such as war or conflict. While the inability to deal with everyday burdens over a period of time may precipitate or escalate a hidden condition, it appears, though, that many Christians, including a significant number of the EGPs I interviewed, think that flouting the biblical command not to worry to a large extent causes emotional/mental illness.[37] Such views may again affect the EGPs' sensitivity in counselling and in any other appropriate response initiatives.

g. Mental illness/distress can be overcome by persons with strong faith and a close relationship with God

The EGPs reflected theologically that the nature of a person's relationship with God and their faith greatly affect their ability to withstand or overcome mental illness, as the following statements suggest:

> The deeper your relationship with God, the more you are able to stand strong, in terms of emotional distress and other things. It is true that you can be shaken, but you won't be moved... *(Rev Tuuli)*

> If the person is matured in faith, he will be able to deal with emotional stress or mental disorder better than a weak Christian or somebody who is a baby in the Lord... *(Rev Osei)*

> ...[i]f the inner man is strong the coping skill of the person is also strong...Yes, if it is there, you might not even get into that state. You may go, but there is a strength that helps. *(Rev Dua)*

From the analysed data, ten EGPs (50%) were emphatic about the importance of a sufferer's level of faith. Reflecting on their views, I also hold that faith in God's ability to deliver or bring a positive outcome from a distressing situation cannot be challenged. In the epistle to the Hebrews, the writer states that 'Without faith, it is impossible to please God'.[38] Indeed, Jesus not only teaches that there are various levels of faith,[39] but also that faith as small 'as a grain of mustard seed' moves mountains.[40] The question to ask is whether the sovereignty of God in determining *how* and *when* He handles a particular situation was also taken into consideration in the EGPs' reflections. Nevertheless, Abraham, the father of faith, kept walking in faith until he received the promised son after twenty-five years, although he may have desired a much quicker answer.[41] Paul's example in 2 Corinthians 12: 7-9 is also an act of faith, demonstrated in his trust in the sufficiency of the grace of God in a seemingly intractable 'thorn-in-the-flesh' situation. Applying the Pauline example in a response to sufferers would also enable them to walk in faith, as they trust, not only that God is *with* them in trouble,[42] but is also able to rescue them from it. It would also encourage them, where recovery is not assured or is delayed, to still trust in God's unfailing love and identification with them through Christ, the Suffering Servant.[43] Therefore, it is for the minister to encourage sufferers and their loved ones to keep faith with God for His healing. As Abboah-Offei declared with conviction, 'I believe Jesus is a healing Jesus. He still heals.'[44] However, Roberts H. Albers and his co-authors imply that it could be insensitive for a pastor to tell persons suffering from mental illness that if only they had faith, or more faith, they would be healed.[45] Two respondents (10%) articulated this point about God's sovereignty and the sufferer's response of trust:

> As we worship God, we cannot say anything bad will not happen. Matthew and other gospels in the Bible say that life's troubles can cause problems for us, but when the problems come, God will relieve or rescue us from them...I think God will one day deliver you from whatever the trouble may be... *(Rev Doku)*

> Worshipping God or being a Christian is about faith. You must have faith that God exists and he can do all things. But after that, as human as we are, we go through some challenges. We believe that God can solve the problem, but even if he fails to solve it, you must still believe that he is God. *(Rev Nsiah)*

I would say in response to Rev Nsiah that God does not 'fail' in solving problems, no matter how dire. It is simply that He chooses His own way and time to solve them according to His wisdom, and in His love and compassion, often in response to the cry of His afflicted children[46] or, as we have discussed above, in response to demonstrated faith.

h. Faith and spirituality used presumptuously or wrongly can have negative consequences

Five EGPs (25%) expressed concern that the presumptuous application of personal faith could cause more harm than good. For instance, Respondent 20, Rev Dua, complained about the congregants' unrealistic expectations, stating that:

> ...[s]ometimes they expect the pastors to pray for the problem to disappear and that is where there is a problem.

For Rev Nanor and Rev Akyia, a sufferer's misapplication of Scripture, stubbornness or state of denial could be the problem:

You are sick, you can't control yourself, you can't even manage the word of God properly... instead of allowing someone to help you, you refuse. Because of your understanding of the Bible, you refuse to even take medicine because they think the word of God will heal them, meanwhile they can't even concentrate well... *(Rev Nanor)*

...[t]here could be situations where some know of the condition they have but may not subject themselves to medical treatment because they think that Scripture says this and that, so they will just believe in God for healing... *(Rev Akyia)*

The issue of Christian sufferers of mental illness not complying with prescribed medication is an important one.[47] According to Dr Ama Edwin, a Clinical Psychologist and Medical Practitioner, it arises primarily from believing they can 'get their act together' by doing more spiritual exercises:

A patient came back to me and she hadn't gotten well. So after two months when she came, she told me she had been fasting. So all the medication I gave her had not been taken...[48]

It appears that sometimes patients are actually encouraged by their pastors and other carers to go off their medication, because continuing is perceived as a sign of weakness. They are told they must have faith for spiritual healing to take place. Edwin expresses her disappointment with some pastors:

[I]nterestingly, I am yet to see someone who ever said they went to see a *jujuman* or *mallam* or fetish person who told them to stop taking their medication... most of the time, pastors are the ones who tell them to stop taking medication... and with some of them, I have been disappointed because these were pastors I knew and I expected better from them...[49]

The distinction that is made between physical and mental illnesses often plays out to the detriment of sufferers. As Michael S. Horton observes, 'If a brother or sister has cancer, diabetes, or a stroke, we pray that God will give the doctors and nurses wisdom and skill to relieve their suffering... And yet, when it comes to mental illness, we still don't really believe that it is a *medical* problem.'[50] This tendency, he says, 'reflects not only a lack of appreciation for the rapid growth in medical diagnosis and treatment of such disorders, but a cluster of theological misunderstandings.'[51]

i. *Faith and spirituality used in combination with community support and other biblical practices has a positive effect*

Five (25%) of the EGP respondents suggested aspects of this sub-theme, which conform to effective models that offer positive outcomes in addition to professional mental help, especially in serious cases of distress. Christian scholars and practitioners who believe in an integrated model of help and recovery often recommend them, as these EGPs advised:

> ...[a]lways be in the company of loved ones. They should also do [their] spiritual exercises regularly and properly through reading the Bible, praying [and meditating] on the Word. They eat well, socialise well and if the person is educated, then read on subjects like that for more information. *(Rev Nanor)*

> ...you [the sufferer] may need one or two matured Christians to get close and help you by using the Word of God and prayer to encourage you and advise you, because when you are in that situation, you tend to forget what God says about that particular situation. *(Rev Mawu)*

> It is not just going there [church] to be prayed for, but do[ing] something meaningful or productive...getting yourself in ministries. All these things help to take away stress. *(Rev Prah)*

Care for the mentally distressed focuses on the body, soul and spirit, and should include devotional exercises such as simple prayer, reading and meditating on the Word of God or listening to audio-taped Scriptures and soothing Gospel music, physical exercising, eating well-balanced diets, socialising with friends, as well as engaging in church activities in ways that enhance one's mental state. It also means having friends and family helping with childcare, marketing or cooking, taking the sufferer to church and the gift of simply being present and listening, just as Job's friends did when they heard of his misfortune. They commiserated with him and sat with him in silence until they resorted to theologising (wrongly) about the cause of his troubles.[52] As Stanford says, 'Little things matter'.[53]

j. *Exercising Christian faith and spirituality is not incompatible with seeking medical help*

Eleven EGPs (55%) were of the view that the use of medical help was not contrary to the Christian faith, but was something they practised in their own ministries:

In the Bible, there were medical doctors who were apostles, someone like Luke. It is never wrong. *(Rev Osei)*

Two EGPs' also emphasised these views:

...[t]hat person should use what the Bible is saying and seek proper attention through medical care or counselling. I think you should also resolve to pray. *(Rev Ntow)*

...[n]ow when people go to church, some refer them to the hospital... When the word of knowledge comes, it brings relief to people spiritually and socially as well. *(Rev Dua)*

These reflections depict, in effect, a certain integration of faith and mental health.

k. *Not all mental illness is caused by demons*

Remarkably, only one EGP (5%) stated emphatically that not all mental illnesses have demonic causes, a fact that the church needs to understand:

I think the first thing they have to do is correct the perception that mental illness is demonic; that causes stigmatisation... I believe as a pastor that not all mental illness is demonic. So, they have to also seek mental treatment and support them emotionally. *(Rev Ntow)*

l. *The mentally distressed are also created by God and must be accepted*

Unconditional acceptance of the emotionally or mentally distressed is not only the basis of all care and support, but is also important if stigma and isolation are to be rooted out. Without acceptance, sufferers of mental illness will always be on the margins, just like the lepers in Old Testament Israel, until Christ came.[54] Some EGPs reflected on the value of sufferers in God's eyes:

...[f]irst of all, they are creations of God; God created them as he created us also. They are blessed; they may have a challenge... *(Rev Anan)*

The pastor is just an ambassador of Jesus, so you have to behave the way Jesus would want. He loves the person; that is why he wants to heal the person... *(Rev Atta)*

Thus, through their theological reflections, all the EGPs attempted to make sense of these experiences and to discern the mind of God on mental and emotional distress and suffering:

I believe that everybody must be treated fairly and equally because they all have the image of God within them. Our professor will say that even the mad man on the road also has an image of God within him, so each person must be treated equally. *(Rev Mawu)*

The EGPs were also consciously or unconsciously making Christian decisions and choices on a matter that emerged from their specific contexts. These choices could be seen in definite acts of acceptance or love:

There was a time we were having a church service and a mental patient came in. Some people were trying to drive him away, but we said, 'No, let him sit down...' *(Rev Bia)*

These reflections thus give rise to the need for fresh insights from the Church to ensure a proper understanding of the issues related to mental illness and distress, as well as the crafting of God-honouring responses towards persons who easily fall into the category of 'the least of these' brothers and sisters of Christ Jesus.

Support of EGPs and Evangelical Churches (E-Churches) for Women's Roles and for Women in Distress

Women's multiple roles and experiences of distress from abuse and violence of all kinds have been identified as major factors in women's mental health challenges. Under this main theme, three sub-themes were identified: i) reliance on women's ministries of churches to support women; ii) pastors' and church leadership initiatives; and iii) pastors' views on what women can or should do to prevent and/or cope with mental ill-health and to improve their wellbeing.

a. *Reliance on women's ministries of churches to support women*

Ten EGPs (50%) indicated that their churches look to their women's ministries or bodies to provide support to women to enable them to handle their expected family and other roles, as well as to help women in distress. As one EGP indicated,

Our women's fellowship is strong here; they give them the necessary information and provide resource persons... *(Rev Dua)*

However, it is also evident from two of the EGPs (10%) on this matter that pastors generally do not show much interest in the actual activities of these women's ministries:

...[i]n our church, we look at these issues through our women's ministry... Pastors do not pay attention to women's ministry. I don't know about your church, but I think it's a general thing. It's cultural too. *(Rev Poku)*

We have a body that is training women, but unfortunately, they don't take the trouble to go. But to some extent, I know they guided them, trained them in some other profession. But to what and extent, I don't know. *(Rev Nanor)*

With one EGP, it appeared that issues of support to women in their roles as wives, mothers, caregivers and in distress are not seen as priority issues or as important as other pastoral responsibilities:
...[i]n our church, our wives take over the women ministry. That is what we encourage them to do. Maybe bigger issues are brought to us, but they meet, share their problems, bring in resource persons and help them. *(Rev Anan)*

In my opinion, the problem here is not so much the work that is done by the often vibrant women's ministries in many churches, nor even the pastors' reliance on them. Rather, it appears that many pastors generally do not take active interest in the women's activities.[55] While not proposing a policing of women's ministry activities by pastors, one would expect the church leadership to be more eager to determine the impact of these activities on members, especially on their general wellbeing, and to ensure that their teachings and activities are well grounded in sound biblical understanding and doctrine.

b.   *Pastors' and church leadership initiatives*
Four EGPs (20%) spoke about the personal sacrifices they made in their ministry to support persons in distress, irrespective of what resources their churches could provide. Respondent 16, Rev Bona, described this aspect of his work:
I have a church outside Wetsa that is dominated by women. Some are widows and others have broken marriages and other things. When I take my allowance, I divide it and give it to them as support because they don't have any money...

Another EGP related his personal initiative as follows:
Apart from marital counselling, I do singles' ministry, especially for young women. Also, post-marital counselling because most of the pressure is on women. I am trying to open up every last Friday of the month for all-night [prayer meeting] to deal with family issues. *(Rev Suni)*

Beyond their personal sacrifices, nine of the EGPs' (45%) said their churches provide financial and other ministry support to their women:

...[t]he church tries to help by giving them financial support where someone wants to start a small business. *(Rev Dua)*

We have a strong women's ministry and their duty is to gather the women [for] training and praying and various aspects of women's issues. They are responsible for themselves, but the church supports them in providing resource persons and the finances in running their various programmes. *(Rev Osei)*

c. *Pastors' views and advice on what women can or should do to prevent and/or to emotional/mental distress or illness*

The EGP respondents had some advice for women on how to protect themselves from emotional/mental distress and illness or how to cope with it. Their focus on women and their relationships was not surprising, since they believed that women's sense of identity is found in relationships with others, particularly men. They also advised against 'church shopping', and the inappropriate use of medicines. Some suggested ways to release stress through godly activities. Some of the extracts below capture the thoughts of the EGPs on women and relationships:

Since most of the women's problems come from men in relationship, they must strictly go by scriptural advice on who (sic) to marry. They shouldn't rush into marriage; after all, it's not a race. *(Rev Nanor)*

They have to understand themselves first...what a woman wants to achieve in life is relationship and what is important to them is their emotions and feelings...So they should know themselves, who they are. *(Rev Ntow)*

...[f]or some of our women, they should not only go with their hearts, but also with their mind when going into relationships. Sometimes you see these things and you tell them and they are not in any way willing to hear the other voice at all; it is not even considered at all. *(Rev Akyia)*

The EGPs who were concerned with what women expected from their churches gave them the following counsel:

...[t]hey must first get involved in the women ministry. They must share their challenges whiles they go there. And, three, get people who are knowledgeable in these areas to always advise, talk and share with them... *(Rev Anan)*

The men of God [in the "one-man" churches] promise women that when they come there, they will get instant solution to their problems. So they prefer going to there instead of mainline churches where God will do his things in his own time. Women should stick to where they are, if it is a God-believing church, and pray. God will listen to them. *(Rev Nsiah)*

On how to handle worry and stress to avoid emotional distress, the EGPs had the following advice for women:

We believe in the biblical teachings and our church service itself involves praises and worship and moments of releasing yourself to God and dancing your stress away... *(Rev Nanor)*

...[w]omen shouldn't get worried. They should put their trust in God, no matter the situation. Also, if it is mental illness, they should stick to the drugs prescribed to them by the physician.*(Rev Bia)*

...[k]now that, as a woman and a Christian for that matter, you always have a second chance before God. So, if something goes wrong now, it doesn't mean that is the end of your life. God can provide. *(Rev Atta)*

In discussing this main theme of EGPs and their churches supporting women in their roles and in distress, the EGPs appeared to have more to say on what women should be and do, than on what they as pastoral caregivers could and should do to support women. While it is evident that the churches are not completely unmindful of the issues that women face which could result in emotional/mental distress or illness, it is equally obvious that pastors could do much more in this area of pastoral ministry to strengthen their work by showing more personal interest, involving the church leadership and providing more resources in initiatives for women.

EGPs' Perspectives on How Evangelical Ghanaian Churches Must Respond
Sixteen of the EGPs (80%) were emphatic about ways they believed churches of the evangelical tradition should broadly address mental health challenges. Even though they felt not enough effort was being made in this matter, their responses however hardly mentioned the possibility of effecting a change through church policy. I discuss the views of the EGPs under the following sub-themes: a) addressing emotional/mental health as part of *Missio Dei*; b) establishing support systems within the churches and for the Church; c)

utilising existing health and other public support systems; d) engaging in awareness, education and training.

a. *Addressing emotional/mental health should be seen as part of Missio Dei*

Of the 20 EGPs, four (20%) were convinced that this was part of the Church's mission. Two of those views are captured below:

> It is a whole ministry, and that was what Christ came to do...*(Rev Awuni)*

> I think the manifesto of Jesus [in] Luke 4:18 says that the Spirit of the Lord is upon me and he has appointed me to give good news to the poor... God is not actually looking at where the problem is but his approach is how to help them out. *(Rev Ntow)*

One EGP) argued that beyond the church, individual Christians could also make it their mission to care for the mentally ill and distressed persons:

> ...[a]part from the church, there is a need for ministries, people who have love for such people and have been educated on such. They should also do some ministry beyond the church to meet the needs of these people. *(Rev Poku)*

Melba Maggay and Haami Chapman point out that rendering loving service in response to human need is one of the marks of global mission. [56] Ministry to persons with mental challenges, I believe, falls squarely under this mark. Indeed, Harold Koenig provides a long list compiled in the United States of faith-based ministries that care for the mentally distressed, set up not only by churches and other religious bodies, but also through individual Christian initiative.[57] Similar initiatives could happen in Ghana as well, when the Church leads the way and encourages its members to pursue such ministry.

b. *Establishing support systems within the churches and for the Church*

Nine EGPs (45%) believed that churches should establish specific support systems such as centres, departments or units to minister to the emotionally or mentally distressed. Two of such views are found below:

> ...[w]e are failing greatly in this aspect. Apart from the prayer and biblical teachings, there should be a special post for helping people with these challenges. This place should be stocked up with qualified people who can both physically and spiritually help... *(Rev Nanor)*

...[g]o the extra mile of establishing rehabilitation centres ...I know that a few churches are doing it, but that is woefully inadequate. I am not sure if there is even any in my church. *(Rev Osei)*

c.   Utilising existing health and other public support systems

One of the EGPs emphasised the need to incorporate such services into already existing church health facilities, while another believed that collaboration with health facilities would bridge the gap:

> We have mission hospitals and other denominations also have them ...We believe in the importance of hospitals and medical treatments for Pentecostal and evangelical believers. *(Rev Doku)*

> I will also say that we need to send them to the hospital. *(Rev Atta)*

c.   Investing in awareness, education and training

Six EGPs (30%) underscored the importance of awareness-raising, education and training for EGPs and the church in order to fundamentally address the issue of inadequate ministry to the emotionally and mentally distressed. Four EGPs (20%) raised the issue of addressing ignorance:

> Are they aware that there is even a problem? First, there must be that awareness that God's creation is being destroyed and other people are on the streets... *(Rev Poku)*

> The Bible says, 'For lack of knowledge, my people are destroyed'. I believe that God wants us to be first and foremost informed about what it is all about. *(Rev Akyia)*

> People come to church and they dance, give offerings and do other things, but emotionally, they are disturbed. It is something that we invest time in...*(Rev Anan)*
> The church too will not like to associate too much with someone who is out of their mind, unless there is somebody who will be there to conscientise them. *(Rev Atta)*

In the EGPs' view, education and training would largely address these concerns:

> I think we all need some general education, because if you are conscious of how to deal with the situation, when it comes, you are able to handle it.   *(Rev Mawu)*

...[p]rovide adequate training not only for the leaders, but to (sic) the entire church. *(Rev Ntow)*

As read previously, the women survivors equally recognised the need for pastors to have a greater knowledge and understanding of these issues. They called for more of them to be educated and trained, not only to guide them in their prayer and decisions for referrals, but probably also to stem their tendencies to over-spiritualise such conditions. It is obvious from the comments above that the EGPs agreed with the women survivors.

EGPs' Perspectives on Formal Collaboration with Professional Mental Health Practitioners

An analysis of the themes emerging from the EGP respondents' data clearly indicates that a majority, that is, 19 (95%) of them firmly believed that the Church and pastors should actively collaborate with professional mental health practitioners (MHPs). Indeed, all 20 EGPs (100%) responded in the affirmative to the question whether they refer people exhibiting mental illness symptoms to professional MHPs. Only one EGP (5%) was indifferent to formal collaboration, even though in his ministry, he referred sick persons to hospital.

The EGPs perceived collaboration in a number of ways: that professionals within churches offer support, or there is actual referral from churches to hospitals or professionals; or integrated teams of pastors and professionals work on cases. The only unidentified model was one where a pastor is also a professional mental health practitioner or where mental health practitioners integrate their Christian faith into their work. The sub-themes that emerged are: a) collaboration is necessary, and b) collaboration must be mutual and useful to sufferers.

a.   *Collaboration is necessary*

For most of the EGPs (95%), collaboration as a form of working together was highly recommended, with the recognition that professional medical or psychological help is important to promote healing:

> We the pastors ourselves, when we are sick and we pray and we are not getting better, we go to the hospital and after two or three injections, we take a rest and continue with the spiritual work. *(Rev Atta)*

Some EGPs believed that collaboration should be mandatory because of the multi-faceted nature of mental health challenges and the need for expertise:

It should not be optional but mandatory, because if you look at it, we work hand in hand. Most issues are either spiritual or medical... What I would take a thousand days praying without results, they can use a few seconds. *(Rev Awuni)*

...[w]e don't have expertise on mental health issues, so when anything like that sets in, it is more advisable to call the experts and we step aside. *(Rev Nanor)*

Still others believed that God sanctions such collaboration:
God has given us these professions to access them. *(Rev Osei)*

It is very good and we need to work together. In fact, it is biblical. As I said, Luke was a medical officer and he worked with the other evangelists... *(Rev Naaba)*

In Evangelist Dr Abboah Offei's opinion, collaboration should have happened 'yesterday'.[58] Not only should the church and professionals consult one another, but holistic healing centres must also be built, where pastors and professionals are found in the same building, working on the human spirit, soul and body at the same time. The single EGP respondent who neither agreed nor disagreed, appeared to have reservations because of the threat of potential 'turf' wars and the desire to forestall the embarrassment of medical professionals' dismissive attitude towards pastors:

I don't disagree with it and neither do I support it... Everyone is important... When it comes to the area of your expertise, you will be able to show your profession. When it comes to my area, I will be able to show my profession... The most important thing is [we] understanding ourselves that we are all useful. *(Rev Akyia)*

This is a legitimate concern, especially in view of the turbulent relationship that has existed between psychological practice and theology/Christian faith. Berinyuu recounts that at the beginning of the 20th century, medical practitioners relegated clergy to the background, even denying them access to their patients.[59] The implications of negotiating such a 'careful marriage' as I prefer to call such collaboration is discussed in the final Chapter.

b. *Collaboration must be mutual and useful to sufferers*
Ten of the EGPs (50%) had in mind mutual and respectful working relationships:

...[i]t should be cordial and constant... *(Rev Awuni)*

The EGPs wanted the services they offered to be recognised as useful and the doctors and medical professionals to also seek their opinion. This would prevent a unidirectional referral process:

It doesn't mean taking the work of the pastor out of his hands. Until that is done, there will be this battle of whether the professional is also becoming a second pastor in the church. *(Rev Tuuli)*

There must be dialogue between the physicians and the pastors so that we are able to draw a clear line between what is spiritual and what is medical. If it is spiritual, the doctors will refer it to ministers who can handle it... *(Rev Mawu)*

...[a] symposium can be organised to draw the line as to what one should be doing in such a situation, because some of the cases are spiritual, and if you are [a] medical person, you can't do anything about it. *(Rev Ntow)*

Abboah-Offei attested to this last perspective. He stated that in the deliverance practice at the Patmos Christian Centre, Akropong, they are able to tell whether a case of someone hearing strange voices is demonic or not. He explained that if it is a medical condition, the person hears the voices in their ear, but if it is demonic, the voices are heard behind their head. Medical professionals could easily diagnose schizophrenia or psychotic depression, when the condition actually required a spiritual response. Abboah-Offei also asserted that even 'spiritual issues have psychological connotations'.[60] These assertions could justify mutual referrals in a properly worked out process of collaboration. Theresa Wiafe-Asante, in her intervention, firmly believed that 'the devil is behind' most illnesses and related two cases where after the interview and prayer, she referred them to MHPs without doing any deliverance. She noted that in both cases, the patients became well after the referral.[61] Dr Akwasi Osei equally assents to fruitful collaboration. He recognises the expertise of pastors in the spiritual field and therefore the need for mutual respect:

Sometimes, the religious practitioners are afraid that if they try to help and the situation gets bad, the medical practitioners insult them when they refer the patients. It should be noted that there are things spiritual people can do which professional MHPs cannot do, especially in the arenas of assurance for simple neuroses and minor symptoms.

Patients want to be assured they are not in grave danger, and this is done very well by Christian healers...[62]

Dr Araba Sefa Dedeh, a Ghanaian clinical psychologist, agrees that MHPs need to collaborate with colleagues in alternative healing to ensure good mental health care and the eradication of practices that may result in the violation of the rights of patients.[63] She adds, though, that more research is necessary for effective collaboration.

Two EGPs (10%) believed that churches could mobilise to take advantage of the existing expertise among their membership for such collaborative efforts. They summed up their thoughts thus:

...[i]f professionals can be grouped in the church and be touched to offer themselves periodically to help churches, it will be good... *(Rev Nanor)*

The pastor and the medical professionals are here, so we should collaborate.
(Rev Awuni)

In conclusion, Mark R. McMinn and Eric L. Johnson both believe that Christianity has much to contribute to psychology, just as psychology to Christian pastoral practice.[64] It is obvious that the EGPs, women respondents, mental health professionals and deliverance practitioners all appear to affirm and support this view. In the final Chapter, I discuss the implications of these findings and make my final assessment on whether the fundamental enquiry of this study has been satisfactorily answered.

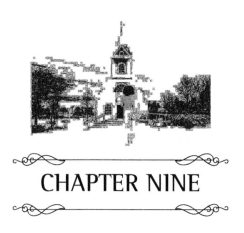

CHAPTER NINE

A CALL TO 'DO JUSTICE AND SHOW MERCY'

Introduction

I began with the proposition that Ghanaian church pastors are a critical and helpful resource for troubled persons, a large proportion of whom are women. Therefore, an evangelical Ghanaian pastor's (EGP's) response to a woman's mental health problem may either help alleviate the problem or further aggravate her condition. In effect, EGPs who are able to recognise and understand the emotional and mental issues of women in their congregations and respond with the appropriate pastoral approaches are likely to obtain positive results for the distressed. In the same vein, I have therefore sought primarily, in this study, to examine whether the African cultural and spiritual worldview of EGPs does not influence how they understand and respond to mental health issues, particularly of women. I have further enquired whether the accusation of EGPs' over-spiritualisation of such distress both in ascertaining causes and in their response is perhaps not due to their cultural and theological understanding of these issues, which in turn leads to a reluctance to complement their practice with medical or mental health resources.

My secondary purpose in this study was to ascertain the emotional and mental challenges experienced by mentally ill and distressed women in order to discern their specific needs as women and to determine any gender differences in causality that may explain their conditions. Following on, would the EGPs understand and take into consideration the appropriate response and help-seeking approaches to adopt in their ministry?

I believe that the findings and results from the analysed data have provided answers to the problem raised. It is crucial that this does not however lead to academic complacency, particularly if the aim of such studies as this present one is to ensure that women in the Christian Church and, indeed, any Christian with emotional or mental health challenges receive the appropriate pastoral responses to their issues. With this in view, I have summarised the significant highlights of my findings and their implications as they emerged. Thus, I hope that the insights I bring to the enquiries raised in the study will be useful for further reflection and my recommendations for a more effective management of mental health in the Church in Ghana will be implemented.

Discussion of Findings and Implications

The first significant issue is the generally accepted belief of a majority of the respondents EGPs, women survivors and the two deliverance ministry practitioners that emotional and mental illness and distress are linked to spiritual causes. The EGPs, also applied mostly spiritual approaches as their first-line response to cases that were brought to their attention. This was hardly surprising because of the African religio-cultural context of all the respondents a context basically primal in outlook and consciousness.

In spite of this strong perception of spiritual causality, however, it is noteworthy that the women respondents appeared not to accept the EGPs' undue spiritualisation of their health conditions because it indicated the EGPs' lack of knowledge and understanding about mental health issues and how to handle such. The findings show that the women did not refuse to be prayed for or to be taken through deliverance sessions. Rather, they were concerned that the EGPs they went to for help did not even suggest they consult professional mental health practitioners (MHPs), much less refer them to MHPs for help. This issue is worth further interrogation, because all twenty EGPs I interviewed stated that they would usually work with, or refer cases to MHPs, when they sensed the need to do so. If the women's experiences of what they perceived as the EGPs' over-spiritualisation are a demonstration of the 'Ghanaian mentality', as one of the women respondents termed it, then it implies that this state of affairs was obviously not satisfactory to the persons being helped. In fact, the women respondents were still able to perceive the over-spiritualisation, irrespective of their conditions of mental ill-health. Since the women belonged to the same religio-cultural context as the EGPs, it is important to heed what they say.

A related issue is that in spite of the over-spiritualisation of causes, the EGPs also ascribed biological, socio-cultural and economic factors to mental conditions, as did many of the women respondents. In one sense, without being wholly conscious of this matter, the respondents were affirming the complexity of emotional and mental distress states and the need to use multi-faceted and multi-disciplinary approaches to both understand and respond appropriately. There is the need, therefore, to go beyond the one-spiritual-solution-fits-all approach to a model that is both culturally sensitive and satisfies the deep religious aspirations of those who minister and those who seek their help.

It is also noteworthy that even though the EGPs proved they could identify conditions of emotional or mental distress in those who came to them, they displayed a profound lack of knowledge of the formal categories of basic mental ill-health conditions. The women respondents on their part firmly believed that EGPs were ignorant in these matters. Most of the EGPs also felt inadequately trained or equipped to handle such cases. While this lack of knowledge did not in any way detract from the critical resources of care the EGP respondents provided to their congregants and those who sought their help, it has implications for their ability to identify symptoms of distress, differentiate in presenting cases, know their limits as well as curbing the tendency to apply more rigorous spiritual exercises to difficult cases. This particular tendency, it must be noted, could result in further burdening the sufferers. As a critical resource, by virtue of their numbers and societal influence, Christian pastors are filling the gap by providing services to the distressed. Their knowledgeability in this arena is therefore essential to ministry.

Another related and important issue involves what the EGPs referred to as 'counselling'. What exactly is the nature of this counselling? How is the therapeutic relationship established in a manner that satisfies the basics of good counselling? If what the EGPs referred to as counselling is not interrogated, the danger is that persons purporting to counsel in Christian churches may do more harm than good. This danger is more real for women especially, because those same relationships built on help-seeking in distress are also fraught with the difficulties of managing transference, male-female sexual tensions and dependency, among other issues. Trained counsellors are presumed to have the capacity to deal with such issues and still achieve some of their counselling goals. Because untrained persons are invariably unaware of these snares, they are likely to fall into them, taking some hapless counsellees along with them. Thus, the need to seriously interrogate counselling as a practice of EGPs' response cannot be overemphasised. Since counselling is therapeutic to the distressed, a good counselling approach is likely to address a significant part of the presenting problem. This should motivate EGPs and the Church to work towards eliminating bad or inappropriate counselling practices from the church. This does not mean, though, that African Christian pastors must necessarily adopt Western models of counselling as 'appropriate' or 'good'. Opoku Onyinah posits that what many pastors practise in their 'prophetic counselling' may be more akin to the Akan traditional practice of Abisa or 'divinatory-consultation'.[1] Abraham Adu Berinyuu also believes that African pastoral counsellors are perceived more as Christian 'diviners'.[2] Both scholars raise important issues that need to be incorporated into developing a curriculum for pastoral education and training in counselling in Ghana. Such inclusion, they reckon, would necessarily take into account the appraisal of African primal concepts and practices with the understanding that primal is not final.[3] Indeed, I maintain that EGPs must pass abisa or 'divination' and other related Ghanaian cultural concepts and practices through the prism of Scripture to discern their light and shade.[4] Whatever holds up under the hermeneutic test of Scripture could then be incorporated into counselling and other therapeutic education and practice. Conversely, whatever is inconsistent must be discarded. Similarly, I propose that some Western psychological concepts and practices in counselling need to be appraised and tested. I will return to this later in my reflections.

One of the major highlights of the findings was the discovery that the EGPs' responses and ministry practices were not based on gender considerations. This was reflected in their actions and not in their perceptions. Indeed, the data did not suggest that they did anything different with women prayer, deliverance, counselling and so on from what they would have done in ministering to men. Neither did they do anything that suggested discrimination or stereotyping. This finding is somewhat surprising as it comes against the background of the EGPs' perceptions of women that conform to strongly gendered societal perceptions of women's 'inherent weaknesses'.[5] The remit of this study did not however allow for a more extensive investigation of this apparent inconsistency between their perceptions and their actual behaviour. A wider study may help ascertain the presence of any marked gender differences in the response to individual cases of emotional and mental distress among EGPs and other leaders in the wider church community.

The EGPs were not against collaboration with MHPs. In fact, the women respondents also seemed to desire this, judging from their answers. They appeared to be aggrieved that they had had to seek professional medical/ psychological help themselves without the involvement of their spiritual help-givers. The common response was, 'None of them asked me to go to the hospital...' Their pastors' silence on this matter may have led to a crisis of suspicion about the MHPs and available resources. 'They always struggle between spiritual solution and medicine, as for that one, they always struggle...', one woman respondent stated. If all the EGP respondents in this study stated that they referred cases to MHPs, yet the women survivors perceived a reluctance on the part of those they consulted, it becomes imperative then that common ground be found to resolve these issues through honest dialogue involving the church, mental ill-health survivors and MHPs. Just because the women respondents expressed a desire for better collaboration between the EGPs and MHPs, it cannot be assumed that this is actually happening, or that it would automatically work out without any challenges. Indeed, a greater integration of mental health knowledge and understanding in the practice of EGPs, as well as the aspiration of MHPs to work towards an integration of faith and spirituality into mental health practice, can only be achieved with greater effort and expectation. Significantly, though, the how of an effective collaboration did not come out clearly in the EGPs' answers, except that most of them preferred a bidirectional referral process that ensured mutual respect between the EGPs and MHPs. I have outlined further in the chapter some recommendations for a possible initiative of collaboration and integration.

REFLECTIONS

EGPs cannot Recognise and Respond to Women's Mental Health Issues without Understanding Mental Health Generally

Reflecting on the insights and lessons from both the literary sources and the data, I realised that women's mental health issues cannot be understood outside the broader questions of mental health. This is because women's emotional and mental health issues stem from our common humanity with all its strengths and weaknesses and from our interaction with others, culture, the environment and God the Creator. Therefore, for the Church and its pastors to gain an understanding of women's mental health issues, they must go back to ask the basic questions: 'What is all this about?' 'How does it affect us as human beings male and female created in the image of God, but broken because of sin and its effects?' 'How does mental ill-health affect me as a person?' 'What does it mean to me as a minister of God, ministering to hurting people?' and 'What does it mean to the Church's mission?' A search for answers to these basic questions while applying the mind of Christ should lead us to a desire to learn from and to provide a more effective compassionate but knowledge-based ministry to sufferers of mental illness, women and men alike.

In exploring these issues, the fact also emerged of the biological and sociological differences between women and men, even though they are created equal as humans before the Creator and in Christ.[6] Again, a search for answers would reveal that these biological and sociological differences have implications for emotional and mental wellbeing or distress in both women and men. Further, it becomes evident that the causes, course and treatment of mental distress may take different paths based on sex and gender differences. This awareness may help greatly in the choice of appropriate and effective approaches to identify and respond to such cases. In effect, EGPs need to know about and understand mental health issues. They also need to understand which women's mental health issues are similar to or different from men's mental health issues, particularly in their interaction with the African socio-cultural and religious context. This understanding is imperative especially because more women than men seek the help of EGPs.

The Story of Two Women: Trusting that God is in the Process of Cure, Healing and Wholeness

Ecclesiastes 11:5 captures succinctly the idea of the sovereignty of God over His creation and in the unveiling of His purposes. The writer cautions: 'As you do not know what is the way of the wind, or how bones grow in the womb of her who is with child, so you do not know the works of God who makes everything.' The suspicion that exists between Christian faith and theology, on the one hand, and psychology as a discipline, on the other, has lasted for several decades and may not be completely resolved in the near future. However, the real life story of two women helps us reflect, not only on the unprofitable artificial distinction Christians make between treatment for physical illnesses and treatment for mental distress, but also on the need to subject it to a thorough theological appraisal. Just as Christians and pastors 'do not know how bones grow in the womb', so should humility and sobriety accompany our understanding of God's sovereignty, as well as His ways of bringing healing and restoration.

In the first story, Adwoa (not her real name), an ardent Christian woman, was diagnosed with breast cancer in her early fifties. She sought the face of God and the counsel of her pastors (EGPs) on what to do: whether to expect direct healing from God through prayer or to go for medical treatment. Before long, her pastors were convinced that she should seek medical treatment as they continued to pray with her. After assessing her situation and the kind of treatment she required, she felt convinced within herself to seek medical treatment abroad. She had little money, so everything that happened for her to travel abroad and receive medical care leading to recovery was nothing short of miraculous. She went through successful surgery and received good after-care from relatives abroad. After her return to Ghana, she discovered the potency of fresh fruits and herbs for cancer recovery. Everyone who knows Adwoa's case is convinced that the hand of God was with her.

Kabuke's story is also that of a serious Christian woman, having come to saving faith in her youth. In her mid-twenties, she was confronted with severe psychological distress. While she prayed and fasted, she also sought the help of several pastors (EGPs) who prayed with her, counselled her and took her through deliverance sessions. However, none of them suggested that she should see a doctor or a mental health practitioner. Rather, they told her she was being 'spiritually attacked' because of a family trait. After several years of this unrelenting 'wilderness' experience, Kabuke suffered a more severe 'attack' in her late forties. She decided then to see a clinical psychologist. During the consultation, the psychologist requested she talk to another woman with similar severe symptoms who had found respite from her research and subsequent therapy. Kabuke did as requested. Within eighteen months, her most troublesome symptoms all but disappeared. She bonded well with her new friend: they prayed together, took their medication, read books on their condition and applied the knowledge to their situation, attended seminars on mental health and supported each other through their painful moments. Today, Kabuke is largely free from the disorder and is living a productive life managing a family, a Christian ministry and a high-powered job.

Some persons have no trouble seeking medical help for physical diseases, but would do everything to dissuade a mental distress sufferer from accessing mental health resources such as medicine, therapy or both. My response to them is to ask: Can they honestly say God's sovereign power to heal and restore was present in Adwoa's case, but absent in Kabuke's? Did God hear Kabuke's every groan and see her every tear? Were their individual decisions divinely inspired or led? If the pastors who counselled Adwoa were the same who sought to help Kabuke, would they have told Kabuke to seek psychiatric help? An honest answer to these questions would probably take care of the internal struggles that Christians and pastors face when confronting similar situations that require theologically sound thinking and practical response. As Matthew Stanford opines,

> Prayer is powerful and transforming because we have a God who hears and responds...In ministering to them, don't make the mistake of saying or implying that all they need to be healed is to pray more or to deepen their faith... each time we struggle with illness or weakness is an opportunity 'that the works of God might be displayed' (John 9:1-3) ... Since our call is to make disciples of all nations (Matthew 28:19), why do we behave any differently towards the mentally ill?[7]

For these two African Christian women, God who knows all things and makes all things possible was glorified. Whether the help they received was physical or mental, each of them acknowledged and expressed gratitude for the role of their care-givers family, friends, doctors, therapists and pastors and for the resources that were made available to them. As far as they were concerned, Jesus Christ worked it all out in His providence, since every stage of the process of their restoration was under His control. These women would probably view their experience through the lenses of Mercy Amba Oduyoye and Elizabeth Amoah and echo what they say:

> The Christ whom African women worship, honor, and depend on is the victorious Christ, knowing that evil is a reality. Death and life-denying forces are the experience of women, and so Christ, who countered these forces and who gave back her child to the widow of Nain, is the African woman's Christ.[8]

Over-spiritualisation, Over-medicalisation and EGPs' Potential Role and Relevant Ministry in an African Context

The African Christian's worldview is that emotional and mental difficulties signify the presence of evil. An analysis of the data established that this thinking leads to the tendency to over-spiritualise distress. Nevertheless, from the same data I have presented views of respondents which suggest that such a one-size-fits-all approach to causality could be detrimental to sufferers because of the complex nature of the pathways of distress. Esther Acolatse critiques the pastoral practices in Africa on the issue of over-spiritualisation.

Acolatse is convinced that African pastors are inadequately equipped to respond to the emotional problems of their congregants. She therefore proposes a re-conceptualisation of the worldview or cosmology that pastors bring to their ministry, which applies aspects of Barthian theology and Jungian psychology as tools for understanding distress and how to respond.[9] For Acolatse, Barthian theology brings the understanding that the human being is 'soul and body undergirded by the Spirit of God' (which He breathed into the body at creation), or in other words, a 'besouled body', undergirded by the Spirit.[10] This new understanding, in Acolatse's view, will help African pastors refrain from spiritualising conditions affecting human emotions, because the spirit of the human being is not like a container within them which can be so affected. Therefore, body-soul (psychosomatic) experiences involving emotions can be effectively dealt with by employing the relevant psychological tools. Acolatse proposes that Carl Jung's psychology on the 'animus', as it affects body-soul interaction and human yearnings that project themselves into distress states, could constitute the re-conceptualised psychological tool.[11] If understood and properly applied by pastors, this tool would not only help the distressed, but would also curb the tendency to use deliverance and similar practices in response to what is perceived as a spiritual problem affecting the *spirit* in a person. In Acolatse's assessment, applying this understanding, while using the proposed tools and emphasising the finished work of Christ in a believer's life and belief in His power over all life's issues, is a more effective way of addressing emotional problems.

On the basis of my own findings, I agree with Acolatse that there is indeed an over-spiritualisation of causes and responses to emotional and mental distress cases. I also agree that African pastors have inadequate training and knowledge of psychological and behavioural sciences, which is a necessary component of pastoral counselling and ministry.

However, I differ with respect to aspects of her proposed solution. The question for me is this: Is it really necessary for African pastors to re-conceptualise their worldview with a Barthian-Jungian approach? It is rather obvious that when it comes to issues of ill-health, and particularly puzzling conditions like emotional or mental distress, the understanding Africans bring from their worldview is that the human being is composed of spirit, soul and body; not compartmentalised, but three composite parts in sync with one another. Whatever goes awry in one affects the others. This worldview is not different from the worldviews portrayed through the Old and New Testaments. Indeed, St Paul prayed that Christians' whole 'spirit, soul and body' be kept blameless at the coming of our Lord Jesus Christ.[12] Many Western Christians, despite the influence of the Enlightenment, also appear to hold the same view of the human being. In effect, Western theologians, scholars, pastoral practitioners, Christian counsellors and psychologists are all seeking to recognise and understand the workings of the human spirit, soul and body, as well as the need to bring healing and restoration to all three in a *holistic* manner.[13] Africans are already involved in this endeavour, except that they apparently place undue emphasis on the troubles and wellbeing of the spirit more than on the other aspects. Thus, if the Old and New Testaments, as well as aspects of Western theological thinking and African concepts are in agreement with one another on the nature of the human being, then there is no need to re-conceptualise the understanding about the spirit, soul and body of the human being.[14] What is required is how to ensure that all components receive the necessary attention in the attempt to bring about healing and restoration through Christian ministry, and as this is being done, emphasise the finished work of Christ in the believer's life.

An interview with Professor Andrew Walls[15] was quite helpful for reflecting on Acolatse's proposed re-conceptualisation and application of the Barthian-Jungian approach. In sum, Walls found Acolatse's work important and useful in its goal of seeking to provide answers to a vital aspect of human existence; that is, by responding to a form of suffering that is not well understood. However, Walls maintains that Barthian theology, like all Western theology since the Enlightenment, is pared down. It is in a sense inadequate to respond to the problem of evil and spiritual realities which African pastors seek to deal with from their own contexts and understanding. He notes that as long as African pastors see such distress states as part of the problem of evil, Western theological frameworks that invariably divorce the spirit realm from the physical, and the sacred from the secular, will not be able to meet the demands of the rest of the world that is more alive to the primal in both consciousness and reality. Walls acknowledges the importance of Acolatse's work also because there is a need for cross-cultural learning Africa and the West need to learn from each other and affect each other's thinking, theology and practices. Indeed, Acolatse herself is aware of this, hence her careful selection of Karl Barth as a Western theologian whose thought bears certain similarities and resonates with the African religious conceptualisation of the human being in relation to God.

In contrast to Acolatse and from my own study, I have come to understand, with specific reference to EGPs,[16] that when they describe a problem as spiritual, it does not necessarily mean that, in all cases, a person's spirit has been possessed or is affected negatively by another spirit or malevolent force. That may be just a part of their thinking. It is also true, though, that to the EGPs, malevolent forces, ill will from others and one's own misdeeds can affect one's body, soul or spirit. In the EGPs' view, a weak faith and personal failure are spiritual issues. The EGPs maintained that any of the composite parts of the being, especially the spirit, if adversely affected, in turn affects the proper working of the other parts. This is what they sought to address and heal with their mostly spiritualised solutions.

Like the EGPs and others mentioned above, I agree with the concept that human beings are spirit, soul and body. When persons are distressed, they *feel* or *experience* its effects on their spiritual lives, even though it may arise from a biological/physical problem, or an emotional or mental state but with no actual impact on their spirit.[17] Thus, a Barthian-Jungian re-conceptualisation may not be necessary as the concept of spirit, soul and body is adequate. What is needed is to frame mental health education or training with content that takes into consideration African Christian religio-cultural sensitivities and aspirations, as well as modern psychological and behavioural sciences. This would enable African pastors to identify and respond much better than they have done to mental health problems, which are often mind/soul-body[18] conditions. No doubt, relevant aspects of Jung's psychology could be included in such a curriculum.

In my view, pastors so trained or educated could play a key role in offering support to distressed persons in such a manner that Richard McNally's concern about over-pathologising their condition and the tendency of applying medical approaches to any and all kinds of distress would be addressed. In other words, when pastors identify emotional and mental issues among their congregants, because they have been trained to do so, they would be able to support persons whose conditions do not need medical or MHP intervention. In addition, even if distressed persons needed such intervention, the pastors would know when to refer them to MHPs, even though their level of support could prevent or minimise strong medical or drug-related interventions. In effect, the pastors' use of a model that integrates the socio-cultural and spiritual needs of the distressed is bound to mitigate the over-medicalisation of Christian sufferers' distress, so that they become a middle way between complaints of over-spiritualisation and over-medicalisation. This is especially important for women because the analysis shows that women are perceived as more vulnerable to emotional and mental distress and illness and in more need of spiritual help in a context that views them as 'weak'.[19] Conversely, literary sources also suggest that women's distresses are more likely to be pathologised and medicalised than men's.[20]

The Bio-Psycho-Socio-Cultural-Spiritual Model: Adopting and Adapting a Framework for Ministry

Having established that the wellbeing or ill-health of one composite part of the human being affects all other parts, and that human beings live in relation to God, other human beings and their environment, one can only conclude that for ministry to troubled persons to be effective, it would need to be approached from this holistic view. This is particularly true for persons with emotional and mental distress or illness. This approach is imperative as one recounts the words of some of the deliverance practitioners I interviewed: '... sometimes emotional issues look like spiritual issues';[21] and '...even spiritual issues have psychological connotations'.[22] Current literary sources from the West are replete with calls to emphasise a holistic multidimensional approach, summed up succinctly by the WHO from the scientific point of view as follows:

> Modern science is discovering that, while it is operationally convenient for purposes of discussion to separate mental health from physical health, this is a fiction created by language. Most 'mental' and 'physical' illnesses are understood to be influenced by a combination of biological, psychological and social factors. Furthermore, thoughts, feelings and behaviour are now acknowledged to have a major

impact on physical health. Conversely, physical health is recognized as considerably influencing mental health and well-being.[23]

The WHO assertion could be said to be only partly accurate, because for the Christian, particularly the African Christian, the Western scientific explanation and model falls short of responding to the soul's yearning for the intervention of the Transcendent God. Biblically, there are several texts that suggest that the attributes God employs to respond to His children when they cry out to Him for help in distress encompass physical, emotional and spiritual protection. Psalm 61:2-5 is an example:

From the ends of the earth I will cry unto You,
When my heart is overwhelmed,
lead me to the rock that is higher than I.
For You have been a shelter for me,
and a strong tower from the enemy.
I will abide in Your tabernacle forever;
I will trust in the shelter of Your wings.

The prophet Elijah encountered God's multi-dimensional ministration during his wilderness flight from Jezebel's threats. He received food, rest, assurance from the 'still small voice', as well as a new assignment.[24] This divine ministration comprised physical, emotional, psychological, spiritual and social components.

Proponents of holistic ministry to the mentally distressed thus appeal for the *bio-psycho-social-spiritual* model to be applied.[25] This model is used at different levels, for example, at the starting point of strengthening Christian theology and faith/psychology dialogue, or while working out collaborative processes between Christian leaders and MHPs, or in integrating mental health into pastoral practices, or for integrating faith and spirituality into formal mental health care practices. However, I have modified this model to include the cultural dimension which is both relevant to the African way of life and context and has implications for mental health and wellbeing, particularly for women. Even within the Western context, the addition of the cultural dimension is vital. The model is thus reframed as the *bio-psycho-socio-cultural-spiritual* model, which I have attempted to capture in the representation below.

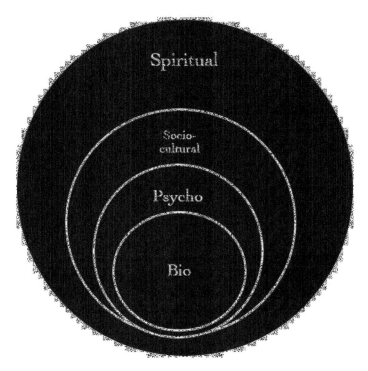

Diagram of the *bio-psycho-socio-cultural-spiritual* model

The above representation shows that the spiritual universe of the African Christian in particular, pervades all things. It is understood and accepted that *Nsɛm nyinaa ne Nyame* (literally in Akan, 'All matters pertain to God', 'God is ruler over all things' or 'God is necessary to all things'). Nevertheless, all other components of the model are recognised as important in and of themselves and as part of the whole, all of which also belongs to God and must be yielded to Him through Christ who 'fills all things in every way'.[26]

With this model, caregivers including pastoral responders, will assess causality from both a holistic and a multidimensional approach, thus applying the same framework for a much more intentional, focused and informed response. Sufferers can also apply this same model in caring for themselves, if possible, and in seeking help from others such as their MHPs or pastors.

Using this model to provide a response or support the distressed believer does not have to be a complicated matter. Nor does it require complex actions. As Stanford notes, 'Little things matter'.[27] The little things could, for example, be as simple as referring the distressed to an MHP and supporting them to take their medicine regularly or taking walks with them in natural surroundings to enhance the psychological component. Other actions to meet their basic social needs may include ensuring that food, shelter and clothing are provided, as well as helping to clean their rooms or wash their clothes. Spiritual needs may be met by praying and studying Scripture with them, picking them up for Church activities and identifying any other needs they or their families may have. Also, responding without judgment to the mentally ill or distressed, while interceding privately for them before the Lord may satisfy the spiritual component of their needs. All these supportive actions could be going on simultaneously throughout the period of the distress.

With women especially, the socio-cultural dimension of explaining distress and response within this framework would mean also paying closer attention to the contextual realities that cause more and different forms of distress to women than men. For example, such helpful actions could be in the form of intervening to negotiate a greater involvement of the mentally distressed woman's spouse and children in house chores and baby care or supporting a woman through the services of a legal aid organisation to get an erring partner to pay maintenance for her children. Similarly, intervention for a widow against maltreatment during and after the funeral period or sheltering a young woman from a forced marriage or other harmful cultural practice are actions that take into consideration the socio-cultural dimensions of women's mental distress.

The Leadership Role of Christian Faith and Theology in Adopting an Integrated Model of Understanding and Response

Ever since the Church Father Tertullian's famous thoughts on the relationship between Athens and Jerusalem,[28] Christians have continued to reflect on the relationship between Christian faith and psychology. My goal is to reflect on what I believe should be the role of the Christian faith in this quest. By faith, I include African Christian theology and its expression of the Christian faith, also bearing in mind that African Christianity can make a dynamic contribution to this quest.

Indeed, as Russel D. Kosits asks, 'Whose Psychology? Which Christianity?',[29] so must African Christians, particularly those of the evangelical persuasion who are the focus of this study, seek to provide scriptural answers to these questions from a perspective that is grounded in Scripture and in the ways that the Gospel engages with our culture. These are not easy questions, but they must be engaged.[30]

Reflecting on this issue, the title of Appiah-Kubi's book, *Man Cures, God Heals,*[31] struck me as instructive, for it sums up what I believe should be the perspective on the contribution of psychology to Christian ministry to the mentally distressed: man cures, but it is God who heals.[32] I would go even further to suggest that man's cure is not outside God's control of and providential care for frail humanity. In fact, for the Christian believer, African or otherwise, God's 'tender mercies are over all His works...'[33] and He superintends every step of the process of healing and recovery for His children. How could man cure, if he is not given the wisdom from above and the resources on earth to use? The question then is this: Are African Christians, aware of our past and primal leanings and now converted, '... turning towards Christ ... everything that is there already, so that Christ comes into the places, thoughts, relationships and world-views in which He has never lived before'?[34] If this understanding of Christian conversion shapes our thinking and practices, then it could be brought to bear on the way psychology could be useful to our Christian ministry. Our faith will lead and shape the ensuing dialogue and practices. Berinyuu succinctly captures this outlook when he states that 'Psychology is relevant but not dominant... Psychology must not dictate to theology.'[35] Echoing the thought encapsulated in Appiah-Kubi's book title, Matthew Stanford, a Western Christian neuroscientist, maintains that 'Psychiatry and psychology offer only symptom relief (which is beneficial), but true hope for recovery and healing is found only in Christ.'[36] In other words, we are called to faith in Jesus Christ, not faith in medical or psychological science. Without Christ, as Edward Mote wrote in his hymn, 'all other ground is sinking sand.'[37]

Thus, concerning religious traditions, Kwame Bediako notes that in the world's disciplines, there are '... indicators which point towards Christ, and there are indicators which point away from Christ.'[38] This is why the discipline of psychology and its practices, beneficial as they are, must go through the same hermeneutic test that Bediako applies to culture. Just as the Gospel is anterior to culture, it is also anterior to all disciplines formulated within culture. Scripture is therefore the hermeneutic of culture and, by implication, of psychology. Even though the benefits of psychology can be applied to ministry, it must be done with the understanding that psychological tools could be used in God's hands to bring relief and some cure to the distressed. African Christians must not only actively engage in this exercise, but should also use the Christian Gospel as 'a precious interpretative key for discerning... what to accept and what to reject.'[39] God is still the God who 'heals the broken-hearted and binds up their wounds.'[40] His process of 'binding up' wounds conjures up a picture of someone gently using a substance on a person's wound to nurse him or her back to health. I consider, therefore, that psychological tools, appropriately discerned, tested through the prism of Scripture, and integrated in response to the needs of the distressed, could represent God's binding work tools in a minister's hands.

Gender-sensitivity in a Ministry to Hurting Women

It is obvious from the data on gendered perceptions that the EGP respondents generally thought of women as emotionally 'weaker' than men, somewhat 'petty' and particularly stubborn in the choice of a marriage partner. It is remarkable, though, that the EGP respondents did not directly accuse any woman of witchcraft in their narration of the cases of women who consulted them, whereas such accusations appear to be common in some churches of different persuasion.

Although the EGPs did not appear to have factored the gendered perceptions in their choices of responding actions, there are other ways they may have subtly or imperceptibly filtered into what the respondents considered as important in pastoral care for their congregations, because of the time and resources they assigned to them. For example, the noted reliance on women's ministries in Ghanaian churches is one of the ways in which women's presence and work, as critical as they are, become marginalised or minimised. In the same ministries, individual women who are facing distress may find support from other women, or feel silenced or condemned, depending on the kind of message conveyed to the membership, particularly if the focus is on the 'idealised' Christian woman who appears to have it all together.

Furthermore, the very nature of the work expected of the women's ministries, I suggest, may invariably increase the burden of women's work. Gender-sensitive ministry to women will therefore help eliminate any stereotyping based on gendered perceptions. It will ensure that women's ministries are not only visible, but the whole congregation is aware of their work. Pastoral care will invariably be directed towards women as individuals without the presumption that the women's ministry would support its own or even that it has the capacity to do so. Gender-sensitive ministry will also ensure that women, men, boys, girls, the aged, disabled, distressed and disadvantaged are all welcome and visible to the shepherd for 'feeding' and 'nurture'.[41]

Gender-sensitive ministry also means an awareness of the peculiar socio-cultural contexts of women that expose them to abuse, harmful traditional practices and marginalisation in decision-making. Its goal is to address such practices within families and the church community. It also goes beyond merely acknowledging the women's life-cycle issues that affect their mental wellbeing to seek ways to protect women from all stereotyping when they are in those stages of life. Of critical importance is the acknowledgment by one of the EGPs that women with problems consult all manner of 'men of God' or prophets, who promise them what they cannot deliver. EGPs perhaps need to refer again to God's admonition to the shepherds of Israel in Ezekiel 34 because they did not strengthen the weak, heal the sick, bind up the broken, nor bring back the straying. As a result, His sheep in Israel were scattered:

> My sheep wandered through all the mountains, and on every high hill; yes, my flock was scattered over the whole face of the earth...became a prey... and food for every beast of the field...[42]

If women, particularly the distressed from EGP congregations, are 'scattering' in search of those who prey on them, then perhaps it is time to focus on how the EGPs and the church can respond in ways that pacify God in His complaint. In the NT, Jesus provides the highest model of gender-sensitive ministry within a patriarchal culture by ensuring the care, visibility and appreciation of women in His time. He responded to them in their full humanity and restored those who sought Him to complete wholeness of spirit, soul and body.

SIGNIFICANT RECOMMENDATIONS FROM RESPONDENTS

The EGPs' recommendations are summed up in three main points. First, the Church needs to see work with the emotionally and mentally distressed as part of God's mission and incorporate it into the Church's mission. Second, EGPs need to be educated and trained in mental health issues, including women's mental health, in order to identify, differentiate and respond appropriately to such cases. Third, the Church and EGPs need to work together with professional MHPs in responding to cases of distress or illness in a manner that ensures mutual respect, bidirectional referrals and inures to the benefit of sufferers.

In their recommendations, the women respondents sought to minimise the over-spiritualisation of their distresses and focused rather on education and training for EGPs on mental health and women's mental health issues. They also asked for collaboration between pastors and professional MHPs as a prelude to better responses and outcomes to their mental health problems.

One of the expert MHPs I interviewed, Dr Akwasi Osei, was emphatic that because the spiritual leaders did certain things better for patients' collaboration was therefore necessary. Dr Ama Edwin, another mental health expert, suggested that collaboration should extend beyond MHPs and the Church to involve all other alternative medicine practitioners in order to ensure regulation, minimisation of fraudulent and dangerous practices and to build capacity for care at all levels. She recommended the enforcement of laws and policies to regulate prayer camps, deliverance practitioners and traditional healing centres, as well as sanctioning those who violate the human rights of the patients.

The two Christian deliverance ministry practitioners I interviewed, Dr Abboah Offei and Theresa Wiafe-Asante also recommended a closer and more structured work relationship between the Christian church and professional MHPs. Both suggested the use of referrals from the Church after assessment and discernment of causality followed by further professional help even after underlying spiritual causes have been dealt with. Dr Abboah Offei went further to recommend the establishment of holistic Christian healing centres, where Christian ministers can work in conjunction with Christian medical and mental health professionals on cases.

MY RECOMMENDATIONS

The focus of this study and the emerging issues may appear to emphasise the pastoral practices of evangelical Ghanaian pastors in particular. However, a key result of the study is that a 'whole' or holistic approach is required when addressing mental health and women's mental health issues. The presence of persons other than pastors is also critical in the help-seeking and healing processes of the distressed. Each sector or person is necessary. Therefore, my recommendations extend to the Government of Ghana, MHPs, the Church, other caregivers and distressed sufferers.

Government of Ghana

The Government of Ghana needs to strengthen the enforcement of the mental health law, policies and plans. This would require that the Mental Health Authority (MHA) monitor all facilities that provide care, whether government or non-governmental. In particular, because abusive practices have been well documented, the MHA would need to closely monitor prayer camps and traditional healing centres in order to stem human rights violations and protect patients from fraudulent practices. The MHA would also need to dialogue with, and dedicate a monitoring unit for, churches and alternative medicine practitioners, as envisaged in the Mental Health Act. This will ensure better regulation of practices and minimise fraudulent practices. For this to be effective, there needs to be an increase in the budgetary allocation to mental health facilities, as well as carrying out an accelerated decentralisation of mental health education and care to community-based facilities. This is particularly important for women facing life-cycle issues such as pregnancy and menopausal care. Thus, midwifery centres and community health posts with their pre- and post-natal facilities could be targeted for support. Funding for mental health research needs a serious boost and any money allocated should also lead to more research on and advocacy for women's mental health.

Another recommendation is the promotion of mental health and women's mental health education through mass media of every kind. In an era of increased incidence of suicides of young women and men, this education cannot be overemphasised. Apart from decentralising mental healthcare, the government needs to ensure that clinical psychologists and other MHPs are posted to regional and district hospitals to facilitate referrals from the communities. The government needs to also recognise the frontline services provided by the Church as part of the mental healthcare response system of the country. With this recognition, the government assumes responsibility for establishing a process of dialogue with the Church and will thus promote, through the design and development of a system of referrals and tracking, a more structured collaboration between professional MHPs and the Church.

Mental Health Professionals

Mental health practitioners (MHPs) have a critical role to provide interview and assessment tools that integrate both cultural and gender-sensitive approaches, including questions about patients' religious beliefs. Ghana's plural religious context may pose some challenges, but the purpose is not to focus solely on patients' religious beliefs and spirituality. Rather, it would facilitate appropriate referrals for the intervention of their spiritual leader, if need be.

Christian MHPs also may establish an active and respectful collaboration with other caregivers, particularly the Christian Church and pastors. Christian MHPs in government service or the churches through their national bodies could initiate a dialogue.[43] This dialogue could form the basis for reaching broad agreements on the processes for collaboration, work relationships, boundaries and ethical considerations. A resource directory of churches, pastors and MHPs could be established at the national and district levels for the purpose of bidirectional referrals.

Finally, MHPs need to work to eliminate physical and verbal abuse of patients in their facilities. Christian MHPs clearly have a role to speak up against such abuses. Also, the Ghana Psychological Council (GPC), the professional regulatory body to which many MHPs belong, would do well to prioritise the training and continuing education of their members. Implementing the law requiring the licensing of all practising counsellors, including those in pastoral counselling, would benefit greatly the churches registered under this body. If the GPC incorporates the *bio-psycho-socio-cultural-spiritual* model into the curriculum for training and education, it would ensure contextual relevance in care and response in mental health.

Caregivers

Apart from pastors, caregivers could include family members, friends, church members and hired health practitioners. It is appropriate, therefore, that caregivers view distressed persons as fully human and accord them all the love, care and respect possible. It is indeed a difficult task to take care of the mentally ill, especially if their condition is complicated or aggravated. It requires much patience and tact. If caregivers educate themselves on the specific symptoms of the disorder, they would be better placed to support the distressed to do all the little things that matter. Such support as getting them to eat well balanced meals, drink plenty of water, take their medication, do their physical and spiritual exercises, meet a doctor's appointment, as well as encouraging them with prayer and Scripture and so on, will all take time, but it pays off in the end.

The caregivers also need to take care of themselves to avoid burn-out or depression. Materials that could be utilised abound on the internet and in books.[44] For caregivers who are not so literate, MHPs who may be part of the team of helpers can provide them with self-care information. To have a friend exercising and holding on to faith on behalf of the mentally distressed is a precious thing. Just as in the example of the four men who brought their sick friend to Jesus through the roof of a house, the faith and prayers of loved ones make a real difference.[45] More important is the gift of presence, as shared by Dr Ama Edwin, who says:

> For those of us who minister to the sick ... I pray that we will tread cautiously when we are privileged to be in the presence of those suffering. No matter their condition we can always give the gift of presence... It's just that; to stay and listen.[46]

The Distressed/Sufferer

It is during the most challenging times of emotional turmoil that staying focused on the promises of God in His word, despite bodily, sensory, or emotional evidence to the contrary, becomes fundamental to the distressed Christian woman or man. If not very ill or when lucid,[47] the distressed person will benefit greatly from reading or listening to Scriptures that point to God's love, comfort, grace, strength, healing and promises of His presence. If very ill, it is enough for the person to remember that he or she is upheld in the 'everlasting arms' of God.[48] Patience with God and oneself is of the utmost importance, because God may also choose to do His work 'little by little' and for a good cause.[49]

Receiving help from others and cooperating as far as possible with one's caregivers, including MHPs, are vital steps to recovery. Treatment may bring discomfort, but avoidance only prolongs distress. Again, for lucid adult sufferers, exercising agency, particularly when making a decision on help-seeking, is important. For example, some women respondents were taken by their family members to places they would rather not have been.[50] This undermines recovery because of potential passive or mental resistance from the sufferer. The resistance could be based on a fear of being forced into a form of syncretism in the quest for healing, an outcome which is counter-productive.

Researching a person's peculiar symptoms is highly recommended. Again, good information abounds if one exercises caution. This brings understanding, reduces the fear of isolation and may be helpful in discussions with MHPs and other caregivers. Alternative therapies that do not 'point away from Christ' are also recommended. These include taking nature walks, keeping a journal, creating artwork, doing simple physical exercises and drinking naturally extracted juice from fruits, herbs and vegetables, among other things. Finally, participation in family and community activities, as well as regular attendance at church services, depending on the person's condition, will be my final recommendation. Emotional and mental illness comes with isolation, whether imposed by oneself or by the society. Even presence and the most insignificant participation in the community of saints is akin to making a prayer of faith and a statement of one's trust in God's presence and help and to God who is present in the gathering of His people.[51]

Christian Women

My primary suggestion to women, like the Christian women survivors who have held on tenaciously to their faith in Christ, is that they do the same in all of life's circumstances. Second, to stay sane and whole, Christian women can learn and work to balance their lives and to consciously take care of themselves, in spite of the societal and family demands on them. This can be done by setting boundaries, negotiating with significant others for delegating tasks and saying 'No' where necessary.

Women need to reach out for help and seek counselling early enough when they are unable to cope well with life's stresses. It is also important that women, especially young women, listen to advice from wise counsellors regarding the choice of romantic and marriage partners since, unfortunately, it is a proven primary source of women's emotional distress.[52]

EGPs and their Churches

The EGPs made recommendations on how to improve their ministry in order to become more responsive towards the needs of the emotionally or mentally distressed, particularly the numerous women who flock to their churches. I have added a few. First, a living relationship with the Triune God that is renewed frequently is vital for ministry, especially for those who provide pastoral care for troubled people.

Second, EGPs do well to know their Scriptures thoroughly and have the hermeneutical tools that enable them to 'rightly divide the word of truth.'[53] This is critical especially for their ministry to the distressed and to avoid the inappropriate use of Scripture. In addition, EGPs need not wait for their church denominations to institute mental health training programmes. In the interim, they can take advantage of Christian health professionals who may be willing to educate them and their congregations. Also, they can take advantage of the many good books that abound with basic information. EGPs can also advocate vigorously for formal theological institutions to incorporate education on mental health and women's mental health into their curriculum and re-training programmes.

Third, EGPs need to make time to train their congregants. This may include organising professional health workers and MHPs in their congregations as resource persons or help-givers. Establishing a programme or department to see to emotional/mental health issues would be commendable. Keeping a database or resource directory of professional Christian practitioners preferred by many EGPs for referrals is also good practice. Finally, Stanford's words are instructive for how pastoral caregivers view their role as vessels in God's hands: '

> ...What you can do is be a part of a process by which God draws you and the other person closer to Himself, transforming you both forever.'[54]

I believe that the African Church has the finest opportunity to test the strength and potential of African theology and Christianity by addressing emotional and mental illness. As Walls observes,

> Theology is about making Christian decisions in critical situations, and it is in the southern continents that those decisions will be the most pressing, and the key theological developments are accordingly to be looked for.[55]

In emotional and mental distress, all the hopes, fears, pains and triumphs of the human spirit exist in a context alive with primal spirituality and the Christian faith. It also provides a testing ground for the maturity or otherwise of African Christianity. If the goal of African Christianity is that Christ emerges from within the world of the African as its only Saviour, then, this is perhaps one of the most critical issues, by the very nature of its complexity, to demand a sound African theological response. Perhaps the poetry of Afua Kuma, the African woman grassroots theologian, may resonate here when she proclaims Christ's triumph over evil and disease in categories of thought from her Ghanaian Akan cultural context.[56] Speaking with conviction from her own personal experiences, she extols Christ's attributes:

> *Yesu na Ɔso kɛntɛn*
> Jesus is carrying a basket
> *Retwe Ɔyaredɔm kogu pobɔn mu*
> Pulling all sicknesses into a sea hole
> *Odu ha bɛfa ɔyare no kɔ*
> He reaches here and takes the illness away
> *Ogyina ɛpo so atee ne nsa*
> He is standing on the sea with hand outstretched
> *Ɔbonsam nenam kwae ase abɔ nnyɛnnyɛn*
> Satan is walking in the forest confused and dazed
> *ɛkoɔ bɔmmɔfo ne amansan boafo,*
> Hunter of the leopard and helper of many
> *Ɔte faako na ɔreyɛ n'awonwannwuma[57]*
> He is sitting at one place doing wondrous works[58]

Like Afua Kuma, the Church has a mandate and a mission to proclaim the power of the risen Christ and the resulting transformation when the Gospel, that is, Christ, encounters culture. Lack of or inadequate attention to emotional and mental distress often keeps Christians in silence, fear and bondage. Freedom comes when the mental illness or distress is brought into the light. Dealing with it under specialised ministries like deliverance may also serve to obfuscate the accompanying but real issues that need to be addressed. Apostle Paul understood this principle of active engagement, as Lucien Legrand points out:

> ...[h]e (Paul) could not stand outside the world he belonged to. It was only from within the cultural complex in which he lived that he could respond to the transforming power of the resurrection and witness to it.[59]

As Paul did, so must the Church. Thus, mainstreaming mental health matters will serve to '...bring every thought into captivity to the obedience of Christ...'[60] when the Church exposes what needs to be healed in the name and power of Jesus Christ, and applies its spiritual arsenal of prayer, deliverance, administering of the Communion, the anointing oil, and other rites, as well as biblically sound pastoral practices to it.

When there is room to discuss, preach about and address emotional and mental distress as one would physical illnesses and other life's challenges, it will also serve to break the stigma and shame people feel about such conditions. Stigma undermines the Church's ministry of reconciliation, peace and justice.[61] Yusufu Turaki insists that, 'Like its Lord, the church must do works of love and mercy and seek justice for everyone, whatever the cost. It must be compassionate in order to hear the cry of the oppressed and the downtrodden and must identify with just and righteous causes.'[62] The Christ who ate with tax collectors and allowed ill-reputed women to touch Him publicly gives the Church the best model for dealing with stigma.

The Church must also be a strong prophetic voice on issues of mental health in the nation. By reason of its caregiving role and substantial influence on large numbers of people, many of whom are national leaders, no other institution is as well placed as the Church to work to eliminate stigma, advocate better funding for mental health services, as well as improve facilities and ethical practice across board. Thus, I fully agree with Howard Clinebell that if the Christian churches 'catch a vision of their potential strength in this area, they can become wellsprings of wholeness and health. What a magnificent opportunity![63]

CONCLUSION

In the 21st century, new questions are emerging from increasingly perplexing situations and issues that require fresh insights and answers from the people of God. God still calls His people to apply their minds to the timeless truths of Scripture, the 'hermeneutic of culture' to bring answers to life's puzzling questions. Mental health and women's mental health issues are not necessarily new issues, but they remain puzzles on the fringes of societal attention. As these issues continue to emerge from specific contexts where complex national socio-political realities interact with global shifts in culture and social relationships, the attempt to apply theology, ideologies, policies and practices to respond to mental health and women's mental health at any level is, to say the least, a daunting task. Yet, the sovereign Lord does not call for a retreat into hopelessness or complacency. He demands a response that continues to demonstrate His presence among His people as the God who gives strength and wisdom, and who challenges His people to seek answers from Him and work toward the transformation of society.

Doing justice, showing mercy[64] and continuing with the task of discipling the nations[65] can answer all these puzzling questions, including the issue of providing loving service in response to the human need of persons with emotional and mental difficulties. Reflecting God's character through the person of the incarnated Christ to those suffering is definitely an ongoing task of Christian mission.

As Christians, our attempt to pool all God-given resources together to respond with the love of Christ towards those who suffer mental illness and distress would hopefully satisfy the cry of the Indian Jesuit cited by Louis Luzbetak:

> You say that you bring Jesus and new humanity to us. But what is this 'new humanity' you are proclaiming? We would like to see it, touch it, taste it, feel it. Jesus must not be just a name, but a reality. Jesus must be illustrated humanly.[66]

This cry echoes that of many survivors and sufferers of emotional and mental distress and illness who reach out for help, seeking kindness and acceptance, as Christ illustrated towards humanity in all its brokenness, not condemnation or withdrawal from other fellow Christians and pastors. The choices we make as the Church of Jesus Christ, to apply all that is good from the resources gifted to us by the Creator, will make a real difference in the quest to minister wholly to those who hurt, be they men or women.

NOTES

Chapter 1

1. In Ghana, there are not enough services to cover the population who require mental health and counselling assistance. See, for example, Human Rights Watch Report, *Like a Death Sentence: Abuses against Persons with Mental Disabilities in Ghana* (USA: Human Rights Watch, 2011).

2. See, for example, Eric L. Johnson, *Psychology and Christianity: Five Views* (Downers Grove, Illinois: InterVarsity Press Academic, 2010), which examines in detail the historically contentious relationship between psychology and religion, particularly Christianity.

3. Andrew F. Walls, 'African Christianity in the History of Religions', in *The Cross-Cultural Process in Christian History* (Maryknoll, New York: Orbis Books, 2002): Chapter 6, especially pages 122-4. See also, Andrew F. Walls, 'Christian Scholarship in Africa in the Twenty-first Century', *Journal of African Christian Thought*, Vol. 4, No. 2 (2001): 48-9. On the use of the word, 'primal', See Andrew F. Walls, *The Missionary Movement in Christian History, Studies in the Transmission of Faith* (T&T Clark: Edinburgh/Maryknoll, New York: Orbis Books, 1996): 120. See also, Kwame Bediako, *Jesus in Africa: The Christian Gospel in African History and Experience* (Yaoundé, Cameroun: Editions Clé/ Akropong, Ghana: Regnum Africa/Glasgow: UK: Bell and Bain Ltd, 2000): 88-9, for an exposition on the 'primal imagination'.

Chapter 2

1. In the modern development of the Church, the Western Church differentiates between Christians of evangelical persuasion and Christians belonging to the Roman Catholic tradition and other denominations that emphasize the supremacy of Church tradition and clergy.

2. In Africa also, there exists an association known as Association of Evangelicals in Africa which was formed in February 1966 at Limuru, Kenya. Its Statement of Faith is similar to that of the USA's National Association of Evangelicals. Four and a half decades after its establishment, it reports that it comprises over 100 million evangelicals, from 36 national evangelical associations and fellowships made up of numerous local churches and para-church organizations. The AEA states that it "... celebrates the diversity of practices and theological emphases

consistent with the AEA Statement of Faith, recognizing the existing dynamic tension between undeniable unity and marvelous diversity." See http://www.aeafrica.org/ , 9th November, 2012, where it defines an evangelical as "someone concerned for the gospel... the Gospel of Christ is central... it is at the centre of his thinking and living."

3. World Health Organization (WHO), Preamble to the Constitution of the World Health Organization as adopted by the International Health Conference, New York, 19-22 June, 1946; entered into force 7 April, 1948, at www.who.int/governance/eb/who-constitution-en.pdf , accessed 25th February, 2016.

4. John Toews, with Eleanor Loewen, *No Longer Alone: Mental Health and the Church* (Waterloo, Ontario: Herald Press, 1995): 15.

5. See, Toews, *No Longer Alone: Mental Health and the Church*: 24.

6. WHO, (2001a), *Strengthening Mental Health Promotion (Fact Sheet No. 220)*, (Geneva, World Health Organization, 2001): 1.

7. American Psychiatric Association (APA), *Diagnostic and Statistical Manual of Mental Disorders*, 4th Edition, DSM-IV (Washington, D.C, USA: American Psychiatric Association, 1994), p. xxi. See, American Psychiatry Association Website at www.psychiatry.org , accessed 3rd March, 2016. See also Joseph W. Ciarrocchi, *A Minister's Handbook of Mental Disorders* (New Jersey: Paulist Press/Integration Books, 1993), p. 4.

8. Vikram Patel, *Where There Is No Psychiatrist: A Mental Health Care Manual* (London: Gaskell/The Royal College of Psychiatrists, 2002): 3.

9. Harold G. Koenig, *Faith and Mental Health: Religious Resources for Healing* (Philadelphia/London: Templeton Foundation Press, 2005): 3.

10. Matthew Stanford, *Grace for the Afflicted: A Clinical and Biblical Perspective of Mental Illness* (Colorado Springs: Biblica Publishing, 2008): 43-44.

11. See for e.g., Koenig, *Faith and Mental Health*: 80.

12. These minor mental ill-health conditions could also be debilitating.

13. See, Toews, *No Longer Alone*: 27.

14. See, Pauline M. Prior, *Gender and Mental Health* (N.Y, USA: University Press, 1999); 4.

15. See, American Psychiatry Association Website at www.psychiatry.org , accessed 3rd March, 2016.

16. For more information on the World Health Organization's (WHO) International Classification of Disease-10 (ICD-10), see, www.who.int/ classifications/icd/en, accessed 3rd March, 2016.

17. Prior, *Gender and Mental Health*: 4.

18. These are broad categories; under each category are several types of related disorders. See summaries of DSM-5 at www.psychiatry.org, and ICD-10 *Classification of Mental and Behavioural Disorders and*

Diagnostic Criteria for Research, at www.who.int/classifications/icd/en/GRNBOOK.pdf, both accessed on 3rd March, 2016. See also, W. Brad Johnson and William L. Johnson, *The Pastor's Guide to Psychological Disorders and Treatments* (USA: The Haworth Press, 2000):7-124; Ciarrocchi, *A Minister's Handbook of Mental Disorders:* 47-178.

19. Vikram Patel, 'Stressed, depressed or bewitched? A Perspective on Mental Health, Culture and Religion', *Development in Practice*, Vol. 5, No. 3, (Aug, 1995): 216-224 (217).

20. Susan G. Kornstein and Anita H. Clayton, *Women's Mental Health: A Comprehensive Textbook* (N.Y: USA: The Guilford Press, 2002): xii.

21. See, Kornstein and Clayton, *Women's Mental Health*: xii.

22. Suzanne Williams, Janet Seed and Adelina Mwau, *Oxfam Gender Training Manual* (UK and Ireland: Oxfam, 1994): 4. Emphasis in the source text. The authors note that the term can meet with resistance among both English speakers and other language speakers because it sounds alien to many people as it is a recently introduced term attempting to bring understanding of the possibility of change in women and men's socially ascribed roles. Being a dynamic term, it shows that gender roles for men and women "vary greatly from one culture to another and from one social group to another. Race, class, economic circumstances, age – all of these influence what is considered appropriate from women and men..." See Williams, Seed and Mwau, *Oxfam Gender Training Manual*: 4.

23. See Work and Family Researchers Network at http://workfamily.sas.upenn.edu/glossary/g/gender-definitions, accessed 23 January 2013. Emphasis is mine.

24. Samuel W. Kunhiyop, *African Christian Theology* (USA/Kenya: HippoBooks/WordAlive/Zondervan, 2012): 1.

25. Kwame Bediako, Lecture Notes, in Master of Arts (M.A) Theology and Mission Class, Akrofi-Christaller Memorial Centre for Mission, Research and Applied Theology (now Akrofi-Christaller Institute), August, 2006.

26. Andrew Walls, *The Cross-Cultural Process in Christian History*: 79.

27. Kwame Bediako, 'Gospel and Culture: Some insights for our time from the experience of the earliest church', *Journal of African Christian Thought*, Vol. 2, No. 2, December, 1999: 8-17, (8).

28. Bediako, 'Gospel and Culture: Some insights for our time from the experience of the earliest church': 8.

29. See, Lena Andary, Yvonne Stolk and Steven Klimidis, *Assessing Mental Health Across Cultures*, (Australia: Australia Academic Press Pty Ltd, 2003), Loc. 831, quoting Draguns, J. G., 'Dilemmas and choices in cross-cultural counselling: The universal versus the culturally distinctive', in P.B. Pedersen, J. D. Draguns, W.J. Lonner & J.E. Trimble (Eds.), *Counselling across Cultures*, (Honolulu: University of Hawaii Press):

3-21 (emphasis mine). See also, Susan Eshun and Regan A.R. Gurung (Eds.), *Culture and Mental Health: Sociocultural Influences, Theory and Practice* (UK: Blackwell Publishing Ltd, 2009): 4.

30. See, for e.g., The Willowbank Report, Report of a Consultation on Gospel and Culture held at Willowbank, Somerset Bridge, Bermuda, 8 – 13 January, 1978: 6 on the features of culture.

31. Eshun and Gurung, *Culture and Mental Health*: 4 (emphasis mine). The authors explain further: "Culture is dynamic because some of the beliefs held by members in a culture can change with time. However, the general level of culture stays mostly stable because the individuals change together. The beliefs and attitudes can be implicit, learnt by observation and passed on by word of mouth, or they can be explicit, written down as laws or rules for the group to follow. The most commonly described objective cultural groups consist of grouping by ethnicity, race, sex, and age. There are also many aspects of culture that are more subjective and cannot be seen or linked easily to physical characteristics. For example, nationality, sex/gender, religion, geography also constitute different cultural groups, each with their own set of prescriptions for behavior. Understanding the dynamic interplay of cultural forces acting on us can greatly enhance how we face the world and how we optimize our way of life." See, Eshun and Gurung, *Culture and Mental Health*: 4.

32. Influences include factors such as globalization, education, travel and migration of individuals, families or groups, etc.

33. Emmanuel Y. Lartey, *In Living Colour: An Intercultural Approach to Pastoral Care and Counselling* (UK: Cassell, 1997): 10.

34. See, Andrew Walls, *The Missionary Movement in Christian History*: 120-121.

35. Gillian Bediako, 'Primal Religions and the Christian Faith: Antagonists or Soul-Mates?', *Journal of African Christian Thought*, Vol. 3, No. 1 (June 2006):12,

Chapter 3

1. WHO, 'Gender and Women's mental health', at http://www.who.int/mental_health/prevention/gender_women/en/, accessed 9 February 2016.
2. The concept of 'feminisation of poverty' has been heavily researched by many organisations, especially the United Nations. See, for example, UN Women, 'The Feminization of Poverty', Fact Sheet No. 1 (United Nations Department of Public Information, May, 2000), at www.un.org, accessed 1 March 2016; Marcelo Madeiros and Joana Costa, 'What do we mean by Feminization of Poverty?', *International Poverty Centre*, No. 58, July 2008, at www.ipc-undp.org, accessed 1 March 2016;
3. See, for example, Burt and Hendrick, *Clinical Manual of Women's Mental Health*: 7.
4. S-G 'Women's Mental Health Report': 9-10. There is also a recent study being done on the differences of men and women's brains. See, for example, Michael Price, 'Study finds some significant differences in brains of men and women', *Referred Academic Journal*, 11 April 2017, at http://www.sciencemag.org/news/2017/04/ study-finds-significant-differences-brains-men-and-women, accessed 22 July 2017. For another interesting study on the subject, see also, Louann Brizendine, *The Female Brain* (USA: Harmony Books/Crown Publishing Group, 2006).
5. Burt and Hendrick, *Clinical Manual of Women's Mental Health*: 2. According to the authors, progesterone and estrogen influence brain function and stress response. Estrogen in women has been examined closely for the role it plays in women's psychiatric illness. See also, S-G 'Women's Mental Health Report': 9-10.
6. Kornstein and Clayton, *Women's Mental Health*: xiii.
7. Burt and Hendrick, Clinical Manual of Women's Mental Health: 7.
8. Burt and Hendrick, Clinical Manual of Women's Mental Health: 7.
9. See, for example, Stewart, Rondon, Damiani and Honikman, 'International Psychosocial and systemic issues in women's mental health': 15.
10. Razee, '"Being a Good Woman"': 45.
11. V. de Menil, A. Osei, N. Douptcheva, A.G. Hill, P. Yaro and A. De-Graft Aikins, 'Symptoms of common mental disorders and their correlates among women in Accra, Ghana: A population-based survey', *Ghana Medical School Journal*, Vol. 46, No. 2 (June 2012): 95-103 (96).
12. de Menil, Osei, Douptcheva, Hill, Yaro and De-Graft Aikins,, 'Symptoms of common mental disorders and their correlates': 96.
13. S-G 'Women's Mental Health Report': 10. (Emphasis in the original test).

14. This is an interesting article worth reading as it explores the topic, 'Why Fewer Black Women Commit Suicide'. See the University of Southern California's webpage, Annenberg Media Centre, at http:// www.neontommy.com/news/2014/08/why-black-women-dont-commit-suicide, Annenberg Digital News, accessed 30 August 2016. The article proposes further research into the issue since it has not been established whether it is because Black women are more resilient to lower depression and suicide attempts due to historical slavery or because of their connectedness to religion, especially the Christian faith.

15. Patel, 'Gender in Mental Health Research': 23. See also, Razee, '"Being a Good Woman": 31.

16. Patel, 'Gender in Mental Health Research': 23.

17. Patel, 'Gender in Mental Health Research': 23

18. Patel, 'Gender in Mental Health Research': 23

19. WHO Report (1997), Gender differences in the epidemiology of affective disorders and schizophrenia (Geneva, World Health Organization, 1997), at www.who.int/mental_health/media/en/54.pdf, accessed 30 August 2016.

20. de Menil, Osei, Douptcheva, Hill, Yaro and De-Graft Aikins, 'Symptoms of common mental disorders and their correlates': 96.

21. See D. Tedstone Doherty and Y. Kartalova O'Doherty, 'Gender and self-reported mental health problems: Predicators of help-seeking from a general practitioner', *British Journal of Health Psychology*, Vol. 15, Part 1 (February 2010): 213-28.

22. Patel, 'Gender in Mental Health Research': 23.

23. Patel, 'Gender in Mental Health Research': 23.

24. Patel, 'Gender in Mental Health Research': 23.

25. Pauline M. Prior, *Gender and Mental Health* (New York: New York University Press, 1999): 24.

26. de Menil, Osei, Douptcheva, Hill, Yaro and De-Graft Aikins, 'Symptoms of common mental disorders and their correlates': 95.

27. de Menil, Osei, Douptcheva, Hill, Yaro and De-Graft Aikins, 'Symptoms of common mental disorders and their correlates': 102.

28. See Alison Moultrie and Sharon Kleintjes, 'Women's Mental Health in South Africa', at http://www.hst. org.za/uploads/files/chap21_06.pdf, accessed 15 August 2013.

29. See, Burt and Hendrick, *Clinical Manual of Women's Mental Health*. That is the main thrust of their book.

30. 68   Dora Kohen (ed.), *Oxford Textbook on Women's Mental Health* (N.Y: Oxford University Press Inc., 2010): vi.

31. Kohen, *Oxford Textbook on Women's Mental Health*: vi. For example, the risk of maternal mortality as a bio-social issue is a significant factor in women's mental health in sub-Saharan Africa, but is not the case

in many Western nations. Also, the need to challenge certain religious and spiritual beliefs and practices (psycho-spiritual factors) generally inimical to women's health cannot be ignored in assessing risk factors, treatment and response.

Chapter 4

1. Ofori-Atta et al, 'Common Understanding of Women's Mental Illness in Ghana': 595. The Ofori-Atta study reported thus: 'It emerged that a common phenomenon within Ghanaian society is for young girls who come from poor families to forge relationships with older men who provide them with material goods and money. Many teachers provided first-hand accounts of how this frequently leads to various mental and behavioural problems in young girls.'

2. Ofori-Atta, Cooper, Akpalu, Osei, Doku, Lund, Fisher and the MHAPP Research Project Consortium, 'Common Understanding of Women's Mental Illness in Ghana': 597.

3. de Menil, Osei, Douptcheva, Hill, Yaro and De-Graft Aikins, 'Symptoms of common mental disorders and their correlates among women in Accra, Ghana: 102.

4. Ofori-Atta, Cooper, Akpalu, Osei, Doku, Lund, Fisher and the MHAPP Research Project Consortium, 'Common Understanding of Women's Mental Illness in Ghana': 592.

5. Ofori-Atta, Cooper, Akpalu, Osei, Doku, Lund, Fisher and the MHAPP Research Project Consortium, 'Common Understanding of Women's Mental Illness in Ghana': 592.

6. Ofori-Atta, Cooper, Akpalu, Osei, Doku, Lund, Fisher and the MHAPP Research Project Consortium, 'Common Understanding of Women's Mental Illness in Ghana': 593. See Actionaid, 'Condemned Without Trial: Women and Witchcraft in Ghana' (Accra, Ghana: Actionaid Ghana/ Actionaid International, September 2012): 8, at https://www.actionaid. org.uk/sites/default/files/doc_lib/ghana_report_ single_pages.pdf, accessed 6 July 2016.

7. Field, *Search for Security*: 149.

8. Field, *Search for Security*: 149.

9. Field, *Search for Security*: 150.

10. See Actionaid, 'Condemned Without Trial: Women and Witchcraft in Ghana': 8.

11. For the full study, see Akwasi O. Osei, 'Witchcraft and depression: A study into the psychopathological features of alleged witches', *Ghana Medical Journal*, Vol. 35, No. 3, 2011: 111-115.

12. For a detailed study on the subject, see Opoku Onyinah, 'Akan Witchcraft and the Concept of Exorcism in the Church of Pentecost', A thesis submitted to the University of Birmingham in fulfilment of the requirements for the degree of Doctor of Philosophy (February 2002), at www.http://etheses.bham.ac/uk/1694/1/ Onyinah02.PhD.pdf, accessed 11 December 2014.

Chapter 5

1. Kodjo Senah, 'Coping with the Health Burden of Violence Against Women', in Kathy Cusack and Takyiwaa Manuh (eds.), *The Architecture for Violence Against Women in Ghana* (Accra, Ghana: Gender Studies and Human Rights Documentation Centre, 2009): 286-316 (290).
2. Senah, 'Coping with the Health Burden of Violence Against Women': 292-3.
3. U.M. Read and V.C.K. Doku, 'Mental Health Research in Ghana: A Literature Review', *Ghana Medical Journal*, Vol. 46, No. 2 (June 2012): 29-38 (29), at www.ncbi.nim.nih.gov/pmc/articles/PMC3645145/pdf/ GM14625-0029.pdf, accessed 17 June 2016.
4. V.C.A. Doku, A. Wusu-Takyi and J. Awakame, 'Implementing the Mental Health Act in Ghana: Any Challenges Ahead?', *Ghana Medical Journal*, Vol. 46, No. 4 (December 2012): 241-250 (241), at http:// www.   ghanamedj.org/articles/December2012/Final/20%Mental%20 Health.pdf, accessed 11 February 2015.
5. V. de Menil, A. Osei, N. Douptcheva, A.G. Hill, P. Yaro and A. De-Graft Aikins, 'Symptoms of common mental disorders and their correlates among women in Accra', Ghana: A population-based survey', *Ghana Medical School Journal*, Vol. 46, No. 2 (June 2012): 95-103 (95).

6. Human Rights Watch, *'Like a Death Sentence': Abuses against Persons with Mental Disabilities in Ghana* (USA: Human Rights Watch, 2012): 7. In the absence of empirical data, the WHO estimates that a tenth of a population may suffer from a neuro-psychiatric illness and one percent from severe mental illness. Ghana's current 24 million population makes that 240,000 for those suffering severe mental illness and 2,400,000 for persons with some form of mental illness. See Doku, Wusu-Takyi and Awakame, 'Implementing the Mental Health Act in Ghana': 241.
7. These are the Accra Psychiatric Hospital, the Pantang Hospital (based in Pantang near Accra) and the Ankaful Hospital (based in Ankaful in the Central Region of Ghana).
8. See Emmanuel Adjei, 'Towards A "Healthy" Future for Mental Health

Recordkeeping in Ghana: The Accra Psychiatric Hospital in Focus', *Ghana International Journal of Mental Health*, Vol. 3, No. 1 (2011): 81-97 (86). Interestingly, as a flagship hospital for psychiatric treatment, the Accra Psychiatric Hospital has been 'involved in mental health care for the past 105 years. Founded in 1906 as a 'lunatic' asylum to accommodate 200 patients, the ...Hospital has ceased to function as an asylum for custodial care and grown into an institution with a bed complement of 600 patients. The hospital has become a place for enhancing mental health, and a training centre for undergraduate and postgraduate mental health professionals under the West Africa College of Psychiatrist.' See also, Olivier Fournier, 'The Status of Mental Health Care in Ghana, West Africa and Signs of Progress in the Greater Accra Region", *Berkeley Undergraduate Journal,* Vol. 24, Issue 3, 2011: 9-34 (10), at http://escholarship.org/uc/item /0gp004t3, accessed 17 June 2016. Olivier Fournier writes about the colonial asylum which later became the Accra Psychiatric Hospital: 'The Lunatic Asylum Ordinance of 1888, enacted by the Governor of the Gold Coast, Sir Griffith Edwards, marked the first official patronage to Ghana's mental health services. This ordinance encouraged officials to arrest vagrant "insane people" and place them in a special prison in the capital city of Accra.'

9. Human Rights Watch, 'Like a Death Sentence': 28.
10. See Mental Health Authority Annual Report, 2017 at www.mhaghana.com, accessed 18 January, 2021.
11. Human Rights Watch, *'Like a Death Sentence'*: 8. For more information on the activities of the Mental Health Authority of Ghana and its Annual Reports, see the Authority's website at www.mhagahana,com, accessed January 18, 2021.
12. Human Rights Watch, *'Like a Death Sentence'*: 29. See also, WHO/ Ministry of Health WHO-AIMS Report on Mental Health Systems in Ghana: 11.
13. *Fournier,* 'The Status of Mental Health Care in Ghana': 13.
14. Alth*ough data is changing fast, this is the most current information on the situation in Ghana:*
15. 29 trained psychiatrists nationwide; 167 gazetted counselling psychologist and 107 clinical psychologists; no psychiatric social workers; Psychiatry Hospitals: 1322 beds (includes 15 beds for children and 79 beds for forensic patients); Accra, Kumasi and Tamale Teaching Hospitals have psychiatric wings; 123 Mental Health/Out-Patient Department (OPD) services countrywide; 1 day treatment facility operated by the Catholic Church in Western Region; Seven Community-based psychiatric inpatient units (5 Regional hospitals plus 2 private clinics totalling 120 beds; 112 beds in Community Residential facilities; Community Psychiatric Nurses (CPN) are available in 159 out of 216

Districts; however, mental health in primary health care is still very limited. See, Dr. Erica Dickson, "Therapy and Available Support for Mental Health in Ghana", Paper delivered at a Seminar organized by the Rotary Club of Ghana, October, 9, 2020, Academy of Arts and Science, Accra, Ghana.

16. See Margaret J. Field, *Search for Security* (London, Gt. Britain: Faber and Faber Ltd/William Clowes and Sons Ltd, 1960).

17. Human Rights Watch, *'Like a Death Sentence'*: 8. Human Rights Watch, which studied eight prayer camps in the country, states: 'Spread throughout the country, prayer camps are privately owned Christian religious institutions with roots in the evangelical or Pentecostal denominations established for purposes of prayer, counseling, and spiritual healing, and are involved in various charitable activities. The camps are run by prophets, many of them self-proclaimed. Some of these camps have units where persons with mental disabilities are admitted, and the prophets seek to heal persons with mental disabilities with prayer and traditional methods such as the application of various herbs. The prophets, or pastors, and staff at these camps have virtually no mental health training. Human Rights Watch has not been able to ascertain the number of prayer camps in Ghana, but there is a general belief...that there are several hundred such camps, operating with virtually no government oversight.'

18. See Read and Doku, 'Mental Health Research in Ghana: A Literature Review': 34.

19. *Fournier, 'The Status of Mental Health Care in Ghana, West Africa and Signs of Progress in the Greater Accra Region': 14.*

20. Human Rights Watch, *'Like a Death Sentence'*: 7.

21. Human Rights Watch, *'Like a Death Sentence'*: 60.

22. Human Rights Watch, *'Like a Death Sentence'*: 7.

23. Human Rights Watch, *'Like a Death Sentence'*: 60.

24. Human Rights Watch, *'Like a Death Sentence'*: 59.

25. Human Rights Watch, *'Like a Death Sentence'*: 61.

26. Human Rights Watch, *'Like a Death Sentence'*: 61.

27. See, for example, Human Rights Watch, *'Like a Death Sentence'*: 65, where it is reported from the study that children with multiple disabilities face worse human rights violations.

28. See Allison M. Howell, *The Religious Itinerary of a Ghanaian People: The Kasena and the Christian Gospel* (Ghana, Accra: African Christian Press, 2001): 213, 251. The phenomenon of the 'spirit-child' among the Kasena of the Upper East Region of Ghana is where a child born with even a minor disability may be referred to as a *'chichiru'*, that is, 'a spirit-related being and not a human being'.

29. Mental Health Act, 2012 (Act 846).

30. *UN Convention on the Rights of Persons with Disabilities (CPRD),* adopted 13 December 2006, by GA Res. 61/106 *and entered into force 3 May* 2008. It was ratified by Ghana on 31 July 2012.

31. Natio*nal Redemption Council Decree (NRCD 30), 1972.*

32. *Doku, Wusu-Takyi and Awakame, 'Implementing the Mental Health Act in* Ghana': 241.

33. See *Mental Health Act, 2012 (Act 846). See also, Doku, Wusu-Takyi and Awakame, 'Implementing the Mental Health Act in Ghana': 242.*

34. World Health Organization and Ministry of Health, Ghana, *WHO-AIMS Report on Mental Health System in Ghana* (WHO, Accra Office/Africa Region, 2011: 9.

35. Mental Health Authority of Ghana, See, www.mhaghana.com, accessed 18 January, 2021.

36. For more information about MEHSOG, see http://www.mehsog.org, accessed 22 April 2016.

37. BasicNeeds, *Charting an Economic Revival for People with Mental Illness and Epilepsy:* 17. Other organisations also working in advocacy and support for persons with mental disability are MindFreedom (Ghana), the Ghana Mental Health Association, Alcoholics Anonymous and a few other user-based civil society organisations.

38. For more details of the analysis in the Report, see WHO/Ministry of Health, *WHO-AIMS Report on Mental Health Systems in Ghana:* 28-31. See also, Dickson, "Therapy and Available Support for Mental Health in Ghana", Paper delivered at a Seminar organized by the Rotary Club of Ghana, October, 9, 2020, Academy of Arts and Science, Accra, Ghana where she outlines several of these challenges.

39. See Human Rights Watch, *'Like a Death Sentence':* 38-67.

40. See also, Human Rights Watch, *'Like a Death Sentence':* 82-87.

41. See, for example, *The World Bank, 'Maternal Mortality Ratio (modelled estimate per 100,000 live births, 1990-2015),* at *www. data.worldbank.org, accessed 17 November 2016.*

42. Government of Ghana/Ministry of Gender, Children and Social Protection (GOG/MoGSCP), *National Gender Policy* (Accra, Ghana: Ministry of Gender, Children and Social Protection, 2015): 17.

43. GSS, Ghana Living Standards Survey (GLSS Round 6), Main Report: xvii.

44. The 2013 overall estimated rate of HIV/AIDS in the country was 1.3%, according to the Ghana AIDS Commission. See GOG/MoGSCP, *National Gender Policy:* 12.

45. GOG/MoGSCP, *National Gender Policy:* 16. See Government of Ghana/ Ministry of Gender, Children and Social Protection (GOG/MoGSCP, 'Gender Statistics in the Republic of Ghana', A Report presented to the CEDAW Conference, Geneva, by the then Minister of Gender, Children

and Social Protection, Nana Oye Lithur (Ghana: GOG/MoGSCP, October 2014). See also, Republic of Ghana/International Development Institute/ Ghana Statistical Service and Associates, *Domestic Violence in Ghana: Incidence, Attitudes, Determinants and Consequences* (UK, Brighton: IDS, 2016).

46. Akosua Adomako Ampofo, Esi Awotwi and Angela Dwamena-Aboagye, 'How the Perpetrators of Violence Against Women and Children Escape: A Study of "escapes" from the time of the Violent Act, through a Formal Complaint, to Prosecution', in Association of African Women for Research and Development (AAWORD), *Women and Violence in Africa/Femmes et Violences en Afrique* (Ouagadougou, Burkina Faso: Cinquième Publication, 2005): 216-250 (231).

47. Ampofo, Awotwi and Dwamena-Aboagye, 'How the Perpetrators of Violence Against Women and Children Escape': 236-241.

48. *Act 29 of 1960 (as amended).*

49. *Act 372 of 2007.*

50. See also, Takyiwaa Manuh and Angela Dwamena-Aboagye, 'Implementing Domestic Violence Legislation in Ghana: The Role of Institutions', in Mulki Al Sharmani (ed.), *Feminist Activism, Women's Rights, and Legal Reform* (London, UK: Zed Books Ltd., 2013): 203-234. For more information on violence against women and girls in Ghana, see also, Dorcas C. Appiah and Kathy Cusack (eds.), *Violence against Women and Children in Ghana* (Ghana, Accra: Gender Studies and Human Rights Documentation Center, 1999); Kathy Cusack and Takyiwa Manuh (eds.), *The Architecture of Violence against Women in Ghana*, (Ghana, Accra: Gender Studies and Human Rights Documentation Center, 2009); Sheila M. Premo, *Coping with Violence Against Women* (Ghana, Accra: Asempa Publishers, 2001); Fiona Leach, Vivian Fiscian, Esme Kadzamira, Eve Lemani and Pamela Machakanja, *An Investigative Study of the Abuse of Girls in African Schools* (UK: Department for International Development (DFID), 2003): 31-68.

51. See Vanessa Brocato and Angela Dwamena-Aboagye (eds.), *Violence Against Women and HIV/AIDS Manual* (Accra, Ghana: The Ark Foundation/Imagine Consult, 2007): 44-51.

52. Ghana Statistical Service (GSS), *Women and Men in Ghana - 2010 Population and Housing Census Report* (Accra, Ghana: Ghana Statistical Service, 2013): 108.

53. GSS 2010 Report, *Women and Men in Ghana*: 108.

54. Osman Mensah, Jody Williams, Richmond Atta-Ankomah and Mboje Mjomba, *Contextual Analysis of the Disability Situation in Ghana* (Accra, Ghana: JMK Consulting, 2008): 31-32, at http://www.gfdgh. org/Context %20analysis.pdf, accessed 23 May 2016.

55. For studies and information on women's status, rights and empowerment

in Ghana, see, for example, Government of Ghana and Ministry of Gender, Children and Social Protection (GOG/MoGSCP), *Ghana's Combined Sixth and Seventh Periodic Reports on the Implementation of the United Nations Convention on the Elimination of all forms of Discrimination Against Women (CEDAW)* (Ghana: Republic of Ghana/MoGSCP, 2011-2015); Ghana Statistical Service (GSS), *Women and Men in Ghana – 2010 Population and Housing Census Report*; Cynthia G. Bowman and Akua Kuenyehia, *Women and Law in Sub-Saharan Africa* (Accra, Ghana: Sedco Publishing, 2003); Kathy Cusack and Takyiwaa Manuh (eds.), *The Architecture for Violence Against Women in Ghana*; Akua Kuenyehia (ed.), *Women and Law in West Africa: Situational Analysis of Some Key Issues Affecting Women* (Accra: Yamen's Printing and Packaging/WaLWA, Faculty of Law, University of Ghana, 1998); and, Christine Oppong, *Middle Class African Marriage* (UK, London: George Allen and Unwin Publishers, 1981), among others.

56. Heather Sipsma, Angela Ofori-Atta, Maureen Canavan, Isaac Osei-Akoto, Christopher Udry and Elizabeth H. Bradley, 'Poor mental health in Ghana: who is at risk?', *Bio Med Central* (The Open Access Publisher, April 2013), at www.https://bmcpublichealth.biomedcentral.com/articles/10.1186/1471-2458-13-288, accessed 17 June 2016.

57. Field, *Search for Security*: 149.

58. *Interview with Dr Akwasi Owusu Osei, Chief Executive Office, Mental Health Authority and Chief Psychiatrist, Accra, 5 April 2016.*

59. Interview with Dr Ama Kyerewaa Edwin, *physician and clinical psychologist, Accra, 5 April 2016.*

60. Read and Doku, 'Mental Health Research in Ghana: A Literature Review': 33.

61. Angela Ofori-Atta, Sarah Cooper, Bright Akpalu, Akwasi Osei, Victor Doku, Crick Lund, Alan Fisher and the MHAPP Research Project Consortium, 'Common Understanding of Women's Mental Illness in Ghana: Results from a Qualitative Study', *International Review of Psychiatry*, Vol. 6, No. 22 (2010): 589-598 (590), at http://r4d.dfid.gov.uk/pdf/outputs/mentalhealth_rpc/ofori-attaetal_intrevpsy2010.pdf, accessed 17 June 2016.

62. Ofori-Atta, Cooper, Akpalu, Osei, Doku, Lund, Fisher and the MHAPP Research Project Consortium, 'Common Understanding of Women's Mental Illness in Ghana': 591.

63. *Ofori-Atta, Cooper, Akpalu, Osei, Doku, Lund, Fisher and the MHAPP Research Project Consortium, 'Common Understanding of Women's Mental Illness in Ghana': 591.*

64. Ofori-Atta, *Cooper, Akpalu, Osei, Doku, Lund, Fisher and the MHAPP Research Project Consortium, 'Common Understanding of Women's Mental Illness in Ghana': 591.*

65.   *Ofori-Atta, Cooper, Akpalu, Osei, Doku, Lund, Fisher and the MHAPP Research Project Consortium, 'Common Understanding of Women's Mental Illness in Ghana': 591.*

66.   Ofori-*Atta, Cooper, Akpalu, Osei, Doku, Lund, Fisher and the MHAPP Research Project Consortium, 'Common Understanding of Women's Mental Illness in Ghana': 592.*

67.   *Ofori-Atta, Cooper, Akpalu, Osei, Doku, Lund, Fisher and the MHAPP Research Project Consortium, 'Common Understanding of Women's Mental Illness in Ghana': 593.*

68.   Ofori-Atta, *Cooper, Akpalu, Osei, Doku, Lund, Fisher and the MHAPP Research Project Consortium, 'Common Understanding of Women's Mental Illness in Ghana': 594.*

69.   *Sipsma, Ofori-Atta, Canava, Osei-Akoto, Udry and Bradley, 'Poor mental health in Ghana: who is at risk?': 7.*

70.   Ofori-Atta et al, *'Common Understanding of Women's Mental Illness in Ghana': 594.*

71.   *Ofori-Atta et al, 'Common Understanding of Women's Mental Illness in Ghana': 595. The Ofori-Atta study reported thus: 'It emerged that a common phenomenon within Ghanaian society is for young girls who come from poor families to forge relationships with older men who provide them with material goods and money. Many teachers provided first-hand accounts of how this frequently leads to various mental and behavioural problems in young girls.'*

72.   Ofori-Atta, Cooper, Akpa*lu, Osei, Doku, Lund, Fisher and the MHAPP Research Project Consortium, 'Common Understanding of Women's Mental Illness in Ghana': 597.*

73.   de Menil, Osei, Douptcheva, Hill, Yaro and De-Graft Aikins, 'Symptoms of common mental disorders and their correlates among women in Accra, Ghana: 102.

74.   O*fori-Atta, Cooper, Akpalu, Osei, Doku, Lund, Fisher and the MHAPP Research Project Consortium, 'Common Understanding of Women's Mental Illness in Ghana': 592.*

75.   Ofori-*Atta, Cooper, Akpalu, Osei, Doku, Lund, Fisher and the MHAPP Research Project Consortium, 'Common Understanding of Women's Mental Illness in Ghana': 592.*

76.   Ofori-Atta, Cooper, Akpalu, Osei, Doku, Lund, Fisher and the MHAPP Research Project Consortium, 'Common Understanding of Women's Mental Illness in Ghana': 593. See Actionaid, 'Condemned Without Trial: Women and Witchcraft in Ghana' (Accra, Ghana: Actionaid Ghana/Actionaid International, September 2012): 8, at https://www. actionaid.org.uk/sites/default/files/doc_lib/ghana_report_single_pages. pdf, accessed 6 July 2016.

77.   Field, *Search for Security*: 149.

78. Field, *Search for Security*: 149.

79. Field, *Search for Security*: 150.

80. See Actionaid, 'Condemned Without Trial: Women and Witchcraft in Ghana': 8.

81. For the full study, see Akwasi O. Osei, 'Witchcraft and depression: A study into the psychopathological features of alleged witches', *Ghana Medical Journal,* Vol. 35, No. 3, 2011: 111-115.

82. For a detailed study on the subject, see Opoku Onyinah, 'Akan Witchcraft and the Concept of Exorcism in the Church of Pentecost', A thesis submitted to the University of Birmingham in fulfilment of the requirements for the degree of Doctor of Philosophy (February 2002), at www.http://etheses.bham.ac/uk/1694/1/ Onyinah02.PhD.pdf, accessed 11 December 2014.

Chapter 6

1. The interviews took place between April 2014 and May 2015.

2. They were all over 18 years old, which is the age of majority in Ghanaian law.

3. Susan Kornstein and Barbara Wojcik, in Susan Kornstein and Anita Clayton (eds.), Women's Mental Health, A Comprehensive Textbook (New York: The Guildford Press, 2002): 151.

4. Angela B. McBride, 'Mental Health Effects of Women's Multiple Roles', American Psychologist, Vol. 45, No. 3 (March 1990): 381-4 (381-2).

5. See A. Ofori-Atta, S. Cooper, B. Akpalu, A. Osei, V. Doku, C. Lund, A. Fisher, and the MHAPP Research Project Consortium, 'Common Understanding of Women's Mental Illness in Ghana: Results from a qualitative study', International Review of Psychiatry, Vol. 6, No. 22 (2010): 589-598, at http://r4d.dfid.gov.uk/pdf/outputs/ mentalhealth_ rpe/ofori-attaetal_intrevpsy2010.pdf, accessed 17 June 2016.

6. Husna Razee, '"Being a Good Woman": Suffering and Distress through the Voice of Women in the Maldives', A thesis submitted in fulfilment of the requirements for the degree of Doctor of Philosophy, School of Public Health and Community Medicine, University of South Wales, Sydney, Australia (August 2006): 91, at http://www.unswork.unsw.edu. au/primo_library /lib-web/, accessed 1 August 2013.

7. Marian J. Alexander and Caitlin McMahon, 'Mental Conditions in Adult Women, Epidemiology and Impact', in Bruce L. Levin and Marian A. Becker (eds.), A Public Health Perspective of Women's Mental Health (New York: Springer Science+ Business Media LLC Publication, 2010): 75.

8. See WHO, The World Health Report 2001: A Public Health Approach

to Mental Health (Geneva: WHO, 2001): 5, at www.whr01_ch1_enWHORep2001.pdf, accessed 22 August 2016. The report states: 'Increasingly, it is becoming clear that mental functioning has a physiological underpinning and is fundamentally inter-connected with physical and social functioning and health outcomes.' An approach to addressing mental illness will take cognisance of the bio/physical, social and psychological factors together. It is important to note that WHO relies on modern information from the fields of neuroscience and behavioural medicine to arrive at such conclusions. The question is how people, sufferers and caregivers alike, from African contexts could make use of such information within their prevailing worldview.

9. See Vikram Patel, 'Gender in Mental Health Research', World Health Organization (WHO) Gender in Mental Health Research Series (2005): 12, at www.who.int/gender/documents/MentalHealthlast2.pdf, accessed 9 February 2016. Patel explains that women are more likely than men to suffer from co-morbid disorders, where co-morbidity is explained as the co-existence of more than one mental disorder.

10. Sheila Walsh, Loved Back to Life: How I Found the Courage to Live Free (Nashville, Tennessee: Nelson Books, 2015): 16.

11. Kathryn Greene-McCreight, Darkness is My Only Companion: A Christian Response to Mental Illness (Grand Rapids, Michigan: Brazos Press, 2006): 105.

12. These churches are popularly classified as 'spiritual churches' or 'sunsum sɔre' in Ghana because of their strong emphasis on the African primal imagination and syncretistic practices. See J. Kwabena Asamoah-Gyadu, 'Drinking from Our Own Wells: The Primal Imagination and Christian Religious Innovation in Contemporary Africa', Journal of African Christian Thought, Vol. 11, No. 2 (December 2008): 34-42 (36).

13. Vivien K. Burt and Victoria C. Hendrick, Clinical Manual of Women's Mental Health (Washington, D.C, USA: American Psychiatric Publishing, Inc., 2005): 170-1.

14. Burt and Hendrick, Clinical Manual of Women's Mental Health: 171.

15. I earlier explained the term sunsum-sɔre and I also refer to the newer independent African churches headed by 'prophets', termed 'neo-prophetism', as distinct from the churches of the Pentecostal-Charismatic movement. Also, as far as possible, I have either omitted the actual names of the churches, prayer centres, pastors and other places or persons, or used letters of the alphabet to represent the churches and prayer centres and pastors, except where use of the names would not have any likely legal implications or where I obtained prior permission to use such.

16. For more detailed discussions, see, for example, Eric L. Johnson, Psychology and Christianity: Five Views (Downers Grove, Illinois:

InterVarsity Press Academic, 2010); Mark, R. McMinn, Psychology, Theology and Spirituality in Christian Counselling (Wheaton, Ill: Tyndale House Publishers, 1996); and David N. Entwistle, Integrative Approaches to Psychology and Christianity: An Introduction to Worldview Issues, Philosophical Foundations, and Models of Integration (Eugene, OR, USA: Wipf and Stock Publishers, 2010). Others are John Toews, No Longer Alone: Mental Health and the Church (Waterloo, Ontario: Herald Press, 1995) and Matthew S. Stanford, Grace for the Afflicted: A Clinical and Biblical Perspective on Mental Illness (Colorado Springs: Biblica Publishing, 2008), among several others.

17. Interview with Dr Akwasi Osei, Chief Psychiatrist, Accra Psychiatric Hospital, Accra, 5 April 2016.
18. 'Florida water' is a form of scented liquid perfume which is thought to have spiritual effects when used in rituals and ceremonies. See https:www.originalbotanica.com/blog/florida-water-uses-ritual-spells, accessed 3 February, 2020.
19. Respondent 2, Akua.
20. Akua and Kaaley (Respondent 10). Kaaley's family represented her at the traditional shrine.
21. This herbalist, whom Rita (Respondent 8) called 'Occult man', used herbs and fragrances and had a shrine where Christian prayers were made. He also called out the 'water-spirits' as part of his treatment. According to the respondent, although his methods reduced her symptoms, he also forced her to have sexual intercourse with him and proceeded to have her family give her to him as a 'wife'. The marriage rites were however never performed. After a number of years, she left him.
22. See, for example, Tedstone Doherty and Kartalova O'Doherty, 'Gender and self-reported mental health problems: predicators of help-seeking from a general practitioner', British Journal of Health Psychology, Vol. 15, Part 1 (February, 2010): 213-228, at www.ncbi.nlu.nih.gov/pmc/articles/pmc2845878/pdf/ulmss-29221.pdf, accessed 9 February 2016.
23. Note that these were not the same pastors randomly selected for this study.
24. Abraham Adu Berinyuu, Pastoral Care to the Sick in Africa: An Approach to Transcultural Pastoral Theology (Hamburg, Germany: Studies in the Intercultural History of Christianity, No. 51; no publication date). Berinyuu calls African clergy or pastors who are consulted by the sick 'Christian diviners'.
25. Esther Acolatse, For Freedom or Bondage? A Critique of African Pastoral Practices (Grand Rapids, Michigan/Cambridge, UK: William B. Eerdmans Publishing Company, 2014).
26. Sarah-Louise Hurst, 'Church leaders' experience of supporting congregants with mental health difficulties', A dissertation submitted in partial fulfilment of the degree of Doctor of Clinical Psychology,

University of Wales, Cardiff and South Wales Doctoral Course in Clinical Psychology, May 2011.

27. Charles Haddon Spurgeon, 'The Valley of the Shadow of Death', original sermon, delivered on 12 August 1880, Metropolitan Tabernacle Pulpit, 1881, Vol. 27: 1595, at http://www.spurgeongems.org/vols25-27/chs 1595.pdf, accessed 4 February 2015.

28. Ian Osborn, Can Christianity Cure Obsessive Compulsive Disorder? (Grand Rapids, MI: Brazos Press, 2008).

29. John Bunyan, Grace Abounding to the Chief of Sinners (first published in 1666), (USA: Evangelical Press, 2000).

30. Chonda Pierce, Laughing in the Dark: A Comedian's Journey through Depression (N.Y, USA: Howard Books, 2007).

31. Kathryn Greene-McCreight, Darkness is My Only Companion: A Christian Response to Mental Illness (Grand Rapids, Michigan: Brazos Press, 2006).

32. Cathy Wield A Thorn in my Mind: Illness, Stigma and the Church (Great Britain, Watford, Herts: Instant Apostle, 2012).

33. Andrew F. Walls, The Cross-Cultural Process in Christian History (Maryknoll, New York: Orbis Books, 2002): 79.

Chapter 7

1. I selected four church denominations that identify themselves as evangelical. I selected these churches out of the many in Ghana because I considered them a fair representation of the range of evangelical denominations in Ghana; from the traditional missionary-instituted mainline evangelical church (PCG), to the older evangelical-Pentecostal denominations, such as the AOG and COP, as well as the more modern evangelical Pentecostal-Charismatic ICGC.

2. Cathy Wield, A Thorn in My Mind: Mental Illness Stigma and the Church (Great Britain: Instant Apostle Publications, 2012). Wield is a Christian, medical doctor and woman survivor of mental illness. She admits that before she suffered a major depressive disorder, she had personally demonstrated stigma in her own attitude towards the mentally ill.

3. Kate Loewenthal, Religion, Culture and Mental Health (UK: Cambridge University Press, 2006): 1-4.

4. Harold Koenig, Faith and Mental Health: Religious Resources for Healing (Philadelphia and London: Templeton Foundation Press, 2005): 39-110. In his discussion of some particular disorders, such as OCD, Koenig acknowledged that in some cases, the symptoms are confused with a person's religious beliefs thereby complicating the disorder.

5. Joseph W. Ciarrocchi, A Minister's Handbook of Mental Disorders (New

Jersey: Paulist Press/Integration Books, 1993): 3.

6. See Vikram Patel, 'Gender in Mental Health Research', World Health Organization (WHO) Gender in Mental Health Research Series (2005), at www.who.int/gender/documents/MentalHealthlast2.pdf, accessed 9 February 2016. See also, WHO, Gender and Women's Mental Health Document, at http://www.who.int/mental_health/ prevention/ genderwomen/en/, accessed February 2016.

7. Interview with Evangelist Dr Ebenezer A. Abboah-Offei, Christian deliverance practitioner, Grace Presbyterian Congregation, Akropong, 21 March 2017.

8. Interview with Mrs. Theresa Wiafe-Asante, Accra, 15 May 2016.

9. Angela Ofori-Atta, Sarah Cooper, Bright Akpalu, Akwasi Osei, Victor Doku, Crick Lund, Alan Fisher and the MHAPP Research Project Consortium;'Common Understanding of Women's Mental Illness in Ghana: Results from a Qualitative Study', International Review of Psychiatry, Vol. 6, No. 22 (2010): 589-598 (590), at http://r4d.dfid.gov. uk/pdf/outputs/mentalhealth_rpc/ofori-atta¬etal_intrevpsy2010.pdf, accessed 17 June 2016.

10. See Richard McNally, What is Mental Illness? (Cambridge, Massachusetts and London: The Belknap Press of Harvard University Press, 2011).

11. Interview with Wiafe-Asante, Accra, 15 May 2016.

12. Interview with Wiafe-Asante, 15 May 2016, Accra.

13. This was extensively discussed in Chapter Four.

14. See Esther Acolatse, For Freedom or Bondage? Critique of African Pastoral Practices (Grand Rapids, Michigan: Willam B. Eerdmans Publishing Co., 2014): 2-11.

15. Matthew S. Stanford and Kandace R. McAlister, 'Perceptions of Serious Mental Illness in a Local Congregation', Journal of Religion, Disability and Health, Vol. 12, No. 2, 2008: 144-153, at http://jrdh, haworthpress. com (doi.10.1080/152289060802/60654), accessed 4 February 2015.

16. Matthew S. Stanford, Grace for the Afflicted: Viewing Mental Illness through the Eyes of Faith (Colorado Springs, USA: Biblica Publishing, 2008).

17. Robert H. Albers, William H. Meller and Steven C. Thurber, Ministry with Persons with Mental Illness and their Families (Minneapolis: Fortress Press, 2012).

18. Marcia Webb, 'Towards a Theology of Mental Health', 2009 Winifred E. Weter Faculty Award Lecture, Seattle Pacific University, 16 April 2009, at http://www.spu.edu/depts/csfd/documents/weter, accessed 23 March 2013.

19. See Vivien K. Burt and Victoria C. Hendrick, Clinical Manual of Women's Mental Health (Washington, D.C, USA: American Psychiatric Publishing, Inc., 2005): 11-40, for an extensive discussion of the connections between women's hormonal changes in menstruation, pregnancy and

menopause
20. See Peter Beresford, 'Social Approaches to Madness and Distress', in Jerry Tew (ed.), Developing Social Models to Understand and Work with Mental Distress (London and Philadelphia: Jessica Kingsley Publishers, 2002): 32-52.
21. See Esther D. Rothblum and Ellen Cole (eds.), Women's Mental Health in Africa (New York: Haworth Press, 1998).

Chapter 8

1. Esther Acolatse, For Freedom or Bondage? Critique of African Pastoral Practices (Grand Rapids, Michigan: William B. Eerdmans Publishing Co., 2014): 4.
2. Abraham A. Berinyuu, Pastoral Care to the Sick in Africa: An Approach to Transcultural Pastoral Theology, (Hamburg, Germany: Studies in the Intercultural History of Christianity, No. 51): 93.
3. Berinyuu, Pastoral Care to the Sick in Africa: 95.
4. The recently established Ghana Psychological Council (GPC) under the Health and Allied Professionals Act, (Act 857), 2013, now requires the registration of all psychologists, therapists and counsellors in Ghana. This includes every pastor who purports to counsel. With this regulation, the requirements of training and certification will be met. The question would then be how training for African pastors would be culturally relevant and sensitive to the contextual realities of persons seeking their help. I must mention that I am a trained Domestic Violence and Child Abuse (DVCA) counsellor, registered with the GPC. I also have basic knowledge in crisis counselling for persons with mental and emotional distress. All the eight or so very kind EGPs I approached for help and encouragement during the period of my personal mental challenges talked with me, but only one took me through a 'talking' process close to what I know basic counselling should offer.
5. Cathy Wield, A Thorn in My Mind: Illness, Stigma and the Church (Great Britain, Watford, Herts: Instant Apostle, 2012): Loc. 2899.
6. See Ian Osborn, Can Christianity Cure Obsessive Compulsive Disorder? (Grand Rapids, USA: Brazos Press, 2008): 129-144.
7. Acolatse, For Freedom or Bondage: 4.
8. Acolatse, For Freedom or Bondage: 18.
9. See, for example, Acolatse, For Freedom or Bondage?: 29. In Acolatse's view, 'The interpretive framework for understanding spiritual phenomenon itself becomes a form of bondage because it completely ignores the aspects of the problems that are purely psychological or physical. When pastors focus diagnosis and remedy almost exclusively

on the spiritual, people suffer unnecessarily, bearing persistent psyche and emotional wounds. When suffering persons do not receive the deliverance they seek, they too often come to believe that they have not received it because of a personal inadequacy. They are convinced either that they do not possess the prerequisite faith or that they may have a hidden sin that blocks the flow of God's healing to them.'

10. Harold K. Koenig, Faith and Mental Health, Religious Resources for Healing (Philadelphia and London, Templeton Foundation Press, 2005: 117. He also maintains that although some patients may show less dramatic manifestations of their illness after exorcism, they continue to be schizophrenic and require medical interventions for their illness.

11. Interview with Mrs. Theresa Wiafe-Asante, Deliverance ministry practitioner, Accra, 15 May 2016.

12. John 16:13.

13. 1 Cor. 12:10.

14. See Human Rights Watch Report, 'Like a Death Sentence': Abuses against Persons with Mental Disabilities in Ghana (USA: Human Rights Watch, 2011).

15. Gary R. Collins, Christian Counseling: A Comprehensive Guide, 3rd Edition (Nashville, Tenn, USA: Thomas Nelson, 2007): 92.

16. Koenig, Faith and Mental Health: 180-181.

17. Gal. 6:2.

18. These sources include Robert Albers, William H. Meller and Steven C. Thurber, Ministry with Persons with Mental Illness and their Families (Minneapolis: Fortress Press, 2012); Matthew S. Stanford, Grace for the Afflicted: Viewing Mental Illness through the Eyes of Faith (Colorado Springs, USA: Biblica Publishing, 2008); John Toews with Eleanor Loewen, No Longer Alone: Mental Health and the Church (Waterloo, Ontario: Herald Press, 1995); Harold Koenig, Faith and Mental Health; Richard V. McCann, The Churches and Mental Health (New York: Basic Books Inc., Publishers, 1962); Paul B. Maves (ed.), Churches and Mental Health ((New York/ London: Charles Scribner and Sons, 1953); and Esther Acolatse, For Freedom or Bondage? Critique of African Pastoral Practices (Grand Rapids, Michigan: William B. Eerdmans Publishing Co., 2014); among others.

19. See, for example, Brad W. Johnson and William L. Johnson, The Pastor's Guide to Psychological Disorders and Treatments (USA: The Hawthorne Press, 2000); Joseph Ciarrocchi, A Minister's Handbook of Mental Disorders, (New York: Integration Books, 1993); and Howard J. Clinebell, The Mental Health Ministry of the Local Church (Nashville, TN: Abingdon Press, 1965, 1972).

20. Koenig, Faith and Mental Health: 3.

21. See the American Psychiatric Association (APA), Diagnostic and Statistical Manual (DSM-5), and the World Health Organization (WHO)

International Classification of Psychiatric Disorders at www.who.int/ classifications /icd/en/GRNBOOK.pdf, accessed 21 August 2016. The APA's latest classification is the DSM-5 (2013). See www.dsm5.org/, accessed 21 August 2016.

22. That is, under the Health and Allied Professionals Act 857 of 2013.

23. Woman Respondent 2, Akua narrated that "[W]hen I finished (eating), they threw the bowl away. Immediately I knew that I was not considered normal. I realized that people do not want to associate with me... that one was really painful to me."

24. See Koenig, Faith and Mental Health: 29. Although the connection between a predominantly Ghanaian Muslim area and the sympathy given to mentally ill persons requires further study, Koenig interestingly notes that among some Islamic communities, the 'insane might be seen as "holy fools" or "wise fools"' and that 'Islamic society had a broad concept of mental illness and was relatively tolerant of deviant behavior.'.

25. John S. Mbiti, African Religions and Philosophy (London: Heinemann Educational Books Ltd, 1989): 166.

26. See Berinyuu, Pastoral Care to the Sick in Africa: 93-108 (100). Berinyuu says that because 'Rituals are an integral part of the practice of the traditional healer/priest and the African life as a whole...', it is a matter of common sense that '...Christian diviners have the task to use all the signs and symbols through which African Christians can believe, feel and experience.' Some of the symbols and rituals he proposes are the use of the rite of anointing the sick with oil, the laying on of hands, as well as the consumption of bread, water and wine. He insists, though, that they should know they have no power in and of themselves to effect change, but it is the work of God's Spirit that makes the difference.

27. See, for example, John Toews and Eleanor Loewen, No Longer Alone: Mental Health and the Church (Waterloo, Ontario: Herald Press, 1995); Paul B. Maves (ed.), Churches and Mental Health ((New York/ London: Charles Scribner and Sons, 1953); Mark R. McMinn, Psychology, Theology and Spirituality in Christian Counselling (Wheaton, Ill: Tyndale House Publishers, 1996); Richard V. McCann., The Churches and Mental Health (New York: Basic Books Inc, Publishers, 1962); and Wayne E. Oates, Religious Factors in Mental Illness (New York: Association Press, 1955).

28. Marcia Webb, 'Towards a Theology of Mental Health', The 2009 Winifred E. Weter Faculty Award Lecture, Seattle Pacific University, 16 April 2009: 34, at http://www.spu.edu/depts/csfd/documents/weter, accessed 23 March 2013.

29. Stanford, Grace for the Afflicted: 240.

30. Stanford, Grace for the Afflicted: 192-5.

31. 'Sakawa' is a contemporary term in Ghana for people who use technology and mystical means to make money or to defraud people.
32. Wilfred A. Agana, 'Succeed Here and In Eternity': The Prosperity Gospel in Ghana (Bern, Switzerland: Peter Lang International Academic Publishers, 2016).
33. J. Kwabena Asamoah-Gyadu, African Charismatics: Current Developments within Independent Indigenous Pentecostalism in Ghana (Leiden: Brill, 2005).
34. John 16:33. Jesus did not minimise trials and troubles in the Christian life, but gave His disciples the hope that He has already 'overcome the world'.
35. Mark 13:34.
36. Hebrews 4:15.
37. In this study, anxiety, as a state of worrying over one's welfare and wellbeing in life which Jesus condemns in the Matthew 6 passage, is to be understood as somewhat different from anxiety as a mental disorder. Some persons with the anxiety disorder may not usually worry over what they will eat, drink or wear. Rather, it pertains to a psychological condition which results in different kinds of phobias and disorders like Panic Disorder, Obsessive-Compulsive Disorder (OCD), Generalised Anxiety Disorder, Asperger's Syndrome and so on. Anxiety can also occur alongside other mental illnesses such as Depression and Bipolar disorder. While it is true that persistent worry over the necessities of life and lack of trust in God's providential care could lead to emotional distress, the debates about the underlying causes of anxiety disorders persist. This issue needs to be explained because many sufferers of anxiety disorders are told they are either 'allowing fear' in their lives, are not trusting God enough, or are being disobedient to the command not to worry or fear. This usually results in more guilt and self-blame in the sufferer. Again, discernment and sensitivity are required on the part of pastoral helpers and other Christians so as not to cause more harm due to a lack of understanding or hasty judgment without a proper assessment. For further explanation, see Stanford, Grace for the Afflicted: 91-109. See also, Dwight L. Carlson, Why Do Christians Shoot Their Wounded? Helping (Not Hurting) Those With Emotional Problems (USA: InterVarsity Press, 1994) and Mitzi VanCleve, Strivings Within –The OCD Christian: Overcoming Doubt in the Storm of Anxiety (USA: Goodreads Inc., 2013).
38. Hebrews 11:6.
39. In the Gospels, Jesus commended 'great faith' (Luke 7:9), but rebuked 'little faith' (Matthew 8:26) and 'no faith' (Mark 4:40) in various disciples.
40. Matthew 17:20.

41. See Genesis 12-21. Abraham and the others commended in Hebrews 11 as heroes of the faith believed God's word, and kept believing, even when they had no evidence of receiving whatever was promised. They were people of faith because they stayed the course, believing God and His Word. Indeed, for many of them, their faith did not keep them out of dangers, afflictions and sorrows (Hebrews 11:35b-39). As the passage teaches, some may not even have been delivered from their dire earthly circumstances because God had provided 'something better' beyond their life on earth (v. 40). Faith demands absolute trust in God irrespective of circumstances and God in His sovereignty honours such faith with reward (Hebrews 11:6b).

42. Isaiah 41:10. See Psalm 91:15. This great and well-loved psalm of God's protection for the believer is recited especially in fearful times. Verse 15 is God's promise of being with believers in trouble to deliver and honour them. That gives comfort to a distressed person.

43. See Hebrews 4:15; 2 Corinthians 4:7-10;

44. Interview with Evangelist Dr Ebenezer A. Abboah-Offei, Akropong, 21 March 2017.

45. See Albers, Meller and Thurber, Ministry with Persons with Mental Illness and Their Families: 21.

46. See, for example, Exodus 3:7-8; Isaiah 49:13.

47. This issue is discussed by Stanford and McAlister, 'Perceptions of Serious Mental Illness in a Local Congregation': 144-153 (151). See also, Stanford, Grace for the Afflicted: 234.

48. Interview with Dr Ama Edwin, Accra, 6 May 2016.

49. Interview with Dr Ama Edwin, Accra, 6 May 2016.

50. Michael S. Horton, 'Faith and Mental Illness', Modern Reformation, Vol. 23, No. 4, July/August 2014:18-25 (18), at http://www.modernreformation.org/default.php?page=articledisplay&var1=ArtRead&var2=1542&var3=main, accessed 5 April 2014.

51. Horton, 'Faith and Mental Illness': 18.

52. See the Book of Job, especially Job 2:11-13.

53. Stanford, Grace for the Afflicted: 232-9.

54. See Albers, Meller and Thurber, Ministry with Persons with Mental Illness: 2-3. In the book, a parallel is drawn between the experience of leprosy and that of mental illness. They write (page 3): 'People who are mentally ill often have the feeling that they are "unclean" and therefore "set apart". They frequently are pejoratively labeled with inhuman epithets, thus spawning inhumane treatment... While most major religious traditions would affirm the inestimable value of human beings, both leprosy and mental illness detract from that precept, resulting in further marginalization and alienation of the sufferer.' Jesus reached out and touched lepers, bringing them healing that was

obviously more than physical (Matthew 8:3; Mark 1:42; Luke 5: 12-13).

55. While there has been little research on women's ministries in Africa and what is available highly commends these groups for their social service to church and community, it may be important to carry out further studies to establish whether some of the women's activities do not actually add to the multiple burdens on women, with implications for their wellbeing. It would therefore be interesting to hear women's voices on this issue. Another question could investigate the content of educating women, especially on what is deemed ideal womanhood: do some of these educational forums affirm Jesus' example of commending Mary for choosing to sit at His feet, rather than Martha's distractions with many activities for His sake? (See Luke 10:38-42.) For a discussion of the immense contributions of women's ministries to the growth of the Church in West Africa in particular, see Ini Dorcas Dah, 'Birifor Women Communicating the Gospel: An Analysis of the Work and Contributions of Birifor Women to the Growth of the Church in West Africa (Burkina Faso, Cote D'Ivoire and Ghana)', A thesis submitted in fulfilment of the degree of Doctor of Philosophy, Akrofi-Christaller Institute of Theology, Mission and Culture, Akropong-Akuapem, Ghana, September 2015. This has since been published: See Ini Dorcas Dah, Women Do More Work than Men: Birifor Women as Change Agents in the Mission and Expansion of the Church in West Africa (Burkina Faso, Cote d'Ivoire, and Ghana) (Oregon, USA: Wipf and Stock, 2018).

56. See Melba Maggay and Haami Chapman, 'To Respond to Human Need by Loving Service (i) and (ii)', in Andrew F. Walls and Cathy Ross (eds.), Mission in the 21st Century: Exploring the Five Marks of Global Mission (Maryknoll, New York: Orbis Books, 2008): 46-61.

57. Koenig, Faith and Mental Health: 157-223.

58. Interview with Evangelist Dr Ebenezer A. Abboah Offei, Akropong, 21 March 2017.

59. Berinyuu, Pastoral Care to the Sick in Africa: 79.

60. Interview with Abboah-Offei, Akropong 21 March 2017.

61. Interview with Wiafe-Asante, Accra, 15 May 2016.

62. Interview with Dr Akwasi Owusu Osei, Accra, 5 April 2016.

63. See Araba Sefa-Dedeh, 'Religion and Psychotherapy', in Angela Ofori-Atta and Samuel Ohene (eds.), Changing Trends in Mental Health Care and Research in Ghana: A Reader of the Department of Psychiatry, University of Ghana Medical School (Accra, Ghana: University Press, 2014).

64. See Eric L. Johnson, Psychology and Christianity: Five Views (Downers Grove, Illinois: InterVarsity Press Academic, 2010): Loc. 342; and Mark R. McMinn, Psychology, Theology and Spirituality in Christian Counselling (Wheaton, Ill: Tyndale House Publishers, 1996).

Chapter 9

1. Opoku Onyinah, 'Akan Witchcraft and the Concept of Exorcism in the Church of Pentecost', A thesis submitted in fulfilment of the requirements for the degree of Doctor of Philosophy, University of Birmingham, Birmingham, UK (February 2002), at www.http://etheses. bham.ac/uk/1694/1/Onyinah02.PhD.pdf: 384-5, accessed 11 December 2014.
2. Abraham Adu Berinyuu, Pastoral Care to the Sick in Africa: An Approach to Transcultural Pastoral Theology, (Hamburg, Germany: Studies in the Intercultural History of Christianity, No. 51, Undated): 93.
3. For a more detailed discussion on the phrase, 'primal is not final', see Gillian Mary Bediako, 'Primal Religion and Christian Faith: Antagonists or Soul Mates?', Journal of African Christian Thought, Vol. 3, No. 1 (June 2006): 12-16.
4. Kwame Bediako, 'Scripture as the hermeneutic of culture and tradition', Journal of African Christian Thought, Vol. 4, No. 1 (June 2001): 2.
5. The women survivors who used the services of prayer camps run by neo-prophets and sunsum sɔre however reported instances of acts of gender-based violence against them, such as witch accusation and physical assault.
6. See Genesis 1:27 and Galatians 3:28.
7. Matthew S. Stanford, Grace for the Afflicted: A Clinical and Biblical Perspective on Mental Illness (Colorado, USA: Biblica Publishing, 2008): 239.
8. Elizabeth Amoah and Mercy Amba Oduyoye, 'The Christ of African Women,' in Virginia Fabella and Mercy Amba Oduyoye, With Passion and Compassion: Third World Women Doing Theology (Maryknoll, New York: Orbis Books, 1990): 35-46 (43).
9. It is beyond the remit of this study to do an in-depth exploration or critique of Acolatse's work on Barth and Jung in all they have to say about the human being and the psyche.
10. See Acolatse's discussion on the nature, components, ordering and differentiation of the human being, in Esther Acolatse, For Freedom or Bondage? Critique of African Pastoral Practices (Grand Rapids, Michigan: William B. Eerdmans Publishing Co., 2014): 90-98.
11. See a detailed discussion in Acolatse, For Freedom or Bondage?: 134-171.
12. 1 Thessalonians 5:23.
13. Berinyuu, Pastoral Care to the Sick in Africa: 83. Author's emphasis. Berinyuu underscores the fact that the influence of Clinical Pastoral Education (CPE) in the United States and United Kingdom is 'also affecting even the scientific treatment of people who are sick. This is

evidenced in the increase in grants for the employment and training of chaplains and renewed interest on the part of governments for the presence of the church in most institutions...' This statement shows that even in so-called secular spaces in the West, the need to minister to the whole of the human person is being increasingly recognised. Anton T. Boison (Boisen) is credited with founding the CPE in the 1920s. It teaches pastoral care to clergy and other spiritual care providers. In Ghana, CPE courses are being offered at a Catholic Diocesan Centre in Koforidua.

14. Andrew Walls, The Missionary Movement in Christian History: Studies in the Transmission of Faith (Maryknoll, New York: Orbis Books, 2009): 120-1. Indeed, the fact that there seems to be agreement between the OT, NT, West and African viewpoints on the spirit, soul and body components of the human being affirms Andrew Walls' statement that '...believers, and for that matter non-believers, are primalists underneath.'

15. Interview with Professor Andrew F. Walls, Emeritus Professor of Liverpool Hope University, United Kingdom and Akrofi-Christaller Institute, Akropong-Akuapem, Ghana, 26 September 2014. Unfortunately, an attempt to reproduce all he had to say would be beyond the remit of this study. Incidentally, Professor Walls also wrote the Foreword to Esther Acolatse's book.

16. I cannot stretch my reflections and conclusions to apply to all African pastors of other Christian persuasions such as the sunsum sɔre and neo-prophetic churches, since my study was limited to only the EGPs.

17. I once had a problem with my spine which, though not painful, produced such distress in my frame that it felt like both a psychological and spiritual issue. Until I was medically diagnosed and understood it, I was convinced that I needed to talk to both my therapist and my pastor. This spine condition is known as cervical spondylosis. The condition may produce anxiety and weird sensations if untreated. When it was medically explained to me, most of the symptoms disappeared.

18. Soul-body conditions are termed 'psychosomatic' in psychology and behavioural science.

19. This is seen especially on TV programmes where it appears that more women in churches are being delivered from all kinds of ailments and attacks, as well as being delivered from being used as agents of malevolent spirits.

20. See, for example, Pauline Prior, Gender and Mental Health (New York, USA: New York University Press, 1999). See also, Cerise Morris, 'Mental Health Matters: Towards a Non-Medicalised Approach to Psychotherapy with Women', Women and Therapy, Vol. 20, No. 3 (1997): 63-77, at http://search.proquest.com/ docview/216249352/ fulltextpdf/1402112D35174B4FC10/1, 26 August 2013.

21. Interview with Mrs. Theresa Wiafe-Asante, Christian deliverance ministry practitioner, Accra, 15 May 2016.

22. Interview with Evangelist Dr Ebenezer A. Abboah-Offei, Christian deliverance ministry practitioner, Akropong, 21 March 2017.

23. WHO, The World Health Report, 2001, New Understanding, New Hope (Geneva: World Health Organization, 2001), at www.who/int/whr/2001/chpt1/en/indexl.html, accessed 22 August 2015.

24. See 1 Kings 19.

25. See, for example, John Toews with Eleanor Loewen, No longer Alone: Mental Health and the Church, (Waterloo, Ontario, USA: Herald Press, 1995): 55-63. See also, Matthew Stanford, Grace for the Afflicted: Viewing Mental Illness through the Eyes of Faith (Colorado Springs, USA: Biblica Publishing House, 2008): 232-3; Robert H. Albers, William H. Meller, Steven C. Thurber, Ministry with Persons with Mental Illness and their Families (Minneapolis: Fortress Press, 2012): 6-7.

26. See Ephesians 1:23.

27. Stanford, Grace for the Afflicted: 231-42.

28. See Tertullien: De Praescriptione Haeriticorum, 7, 9-13 (CCL 1): 193, in Volumes 1 and 11 of Corpus Christianorum, Series Latina (CCL), Turnhout, 1954.

29. Russel D. Kosits, 'Whose Psychology? Which Christianity?', McMaster Journal of Theology and Ministry (MJTM), Vol. 12 (2011-2012): 101-195 (107).Kosits writes: 'Though the Bible tends not to provide the data of psychology, it provides the ultimate framework for the interpretation of the data of psychology, apart from which the psychological science suffers greatly.' He argues for a strong emphasis on the Bible and careful attentiveness to scriptural revelation, in order to stem the replacement of biblical faith and revelation with whatever comes out of the academic establishment. I share this view completely.

30. Even though I propose a model of practice that uses words such as 'collaboration' and 'integration' as part of the interpretive framework of this study, these are still somewhat nebulous terms since academicians, theologians and practitioners do not all have the same understanding of these words. Collaboration, I would concede, is easier to understand in theory and in practice than integration. However, I admit that this is part of the struggle of human existence, and we're all trying to make meaning and sense of the puzzling issues of our times. I can only pray, therefore, that evangelical Christians and the Church will find what I mean to say in these terms clearer and more amenable to application than not, as they engage with the African Christian context. Of course, in the areas of scholarship and practice, this is still unfinished business.

31. Kofi Appiah-Kubi, Man Cures, God Heals: Religion and Medical Practice among the Akan of Ghana (New Jersey, USA: Allanheld, Osmun & Co.,

1981). It is outside the scope of our discussion here to delve into the primary thrust of Appiah-Kubi's book on Akan medical thought and practices in relation to the healthcare system of Ghana.

32. In an interesting discussion on 16 July 2017, Professor Allison Howell reflected further on the statement, 'Man cures, God heals', and asked me whether human beings ever fully succeed in curing illnesses. In her view, there are many illnesses that doctors would say are 'in remission', but not fully cured. She opined that in an imperfect world, it appears that all of life is 'in remission.' To her, it is more truthful to say instead that 'Man treats, God heals.'

33. Psalm 145:9.

34. Andrew F. Walls, 'The Significance of Christianity in Africa', A Lecture given at St Colm (Edinburgh: Church of Scotland/St. Colm's Education Centre and College, 1989): 20. For a similar statement on conversion, see also, Andrew F. Walls, The Missionary Movement in Christian History: Studies in the Transmission of Faith (Maryknoll, New York: Orbis Books, 2009): 28.

35. Berinyuu, Pastoral Care for the Sick in Africa: 85.

36. Stanford, Grace for the Afflicted: 239.

37. The quote is the last line of the refrain of the hymn 'My Hope is Built on Nothing Less' by Edward Mote (1797-1874). It is found in United Methodist Hymnal, No. 368.

38. Kwame Bediako, Jesus in Africa, The Christian Gospel in African History and Experience (UK: Regnum Africa, 2000): 41. The 2013 Tavistock Report from the UK, for example, is very detailed in how alternative practitioners who deal with mental health issues attempt to incorporate many different practices from different traditions and countries to help sufferers. See Dione Hills, E. Aram, D. Hinds, C. Warrington, L. Brisett, L. Stock, 'Traditional Healers Action Research Project', Final Report prepared by the Tavistock Institute of Human Relations (for The King's Fund), London, UK, 13 May 2013: 58-70. In my opinion, this underscores the urgent task of applying the hermeneutical test for healing practices and traditions which may end up being adopted to help in particular Christian sufferers who want to be conformed to Christ and consistent in their Christian beliefs and practices.

39. Bediako, Jesus in Africa: 73.

40. Psalm 147:3.

41. See John 21: 15-17.

42. Ezekiel 34:1-10 (6, 7).

43. These bodies include the Christian Council of Ghana (CCG), the National Association of Charismatic Churches (NACC) and the National Pentecostal Council (NPC).

44. Internet material should be used with discernment and caution because

materials abound that are of questionable sources and content. Using well-established organisational websites with well-researched resources is advised.

45. Mark 2:5 and Luke 5:20. I have been concerned to hear family members of a mentally distressed person say to them that if they had more faith, they would be healed. I have seen how it visibly increases the distress of the sufferer to hear that said. It appears these family members do not think that their own faith may also be lacking if viewed against the background of these Scriptures.

46. Conversation with Dr Ama Edwin, Accra, 8 May 2017.

47. The expression 'lucid' is used here to mean when a person has or shows the ability to think clearly in intervals between periods of mental confusion, distress or illness.

48. Deuteronomy 33:27.

49. Some verses of Scriptures that the distressed Christian could memorise to understand why patience is needed when seeking recovery is Exodus 23:29-30: 'I will not drive them out before thee in one year; lest the land become desolate and the beasts of the field multiply against thee. Little by little, I will drive them out before thee, until thou be increased, and inherit the land.' (KJV)

50. These places included neo-prophetic churches, sunsum sɔre and traditional healing centres.

51. See Psalm 46: 1.

52. At the risk of sounding stereotypical, I have been in counselling long enough to know that the EGPs may be right when they fault some women in that aspect of their lives, once they make up their minds about a marriage partner.

53. 2 Timothy 2:15.

54. Stanford, Grace for the Afflicted: 232.

55. Andrew F. Walls, 'Christian Scholarship in Africa in the Twenty-first Century', Journal of African Christian Thought, Vol. 4, No. 2 (December 2001): 47.

56. Afua Kuma, Kwaeberentuw ase Yesu (Ghana: Asempa Publishers, 1981). See also, Afua Kuma, Jesus of the Deep Forest: Prayers and Praises of Afua Kuma (English Translation by Jon Kirby of Original Twi texts) (Accra: Asempa Publishers, 1981).

57. Kuma, Kwaeberentuw ase Yesu: 32.

58. This is my English translation of the extract in Twi. See Jon Kirby, Jesus of the Deep Forest: Prayers and Praises of Afua Kuma for his English translation.

59. Lucien Legrand, The Bible on Culture (Maryknoll, New York, USA: Orbis Books, 2000): 143.

60. 2 Corinthians 10:5.

61. See 2 Corinthians 5:18-21; Matthew 5:9; and Micah 6:8.

62. Yusufu Turaki, 'Truth, Justice and Reconciliation', in Tokunboh Adeyemo (Gen. ed.), Africa Bible Commentary: A One-Volume Commentary (Africa: Word Alive Publishers/Zondervan, 2008): 875.

63. Howard Clinebell, The Mental Health Ministry of the Local Church (Nashville, New York: Abingdon Press, 1972): 281.

64. Micah 6:8.

65. Matthew 28: 18-20.

66. Louis L. Luzbetak, The Church and Cultures: New Perspectives in Missiological Anthropology (Maryknoll, New York: Orbis Books, 2000): 374.

BIBLIOGRAPHY

Published Books

Acolatse, Esther, *For Freedom or Bondage? A Critique of African Pastoral Practices* (Grand Rapids, Michigan/Cambridge, UK: William B. Eerdmans Publishing Company, 2014).

Adams, Jay, *The Christian Counselor's Manual: The Practice of Nouthetic Counseling* (Grand Rapids, Michigan: Zondervan, 1973).

Adeyemo, Tokunboh (Gen. ed.), *Africa Bible Commentary: A One-Volume Commentary*, (Africa: Word Alive Publishers/Zondervan, 2008).

Agana, Wilfred A., *'Succeed Here and In Eternity: The Prosperity Gospel in Ghana* (Bern, Switzerland: Peter Lang International Academic Publishers, 2016).

Albers, Roberts H., William H. Meller and Steven C. Thurber, *Ministry with Persons with Mental Illness and their Families* (Minneapolis: Fortress Press, 2012).

Andary, Lena, Yvonne Stolk, and Steven Klimidis, *Assessing Mental Health Across Cultures* (Australia: Australia Academic Press Pty. Ltd, 2003).

Asamoah-Gyadu, Kwabena, *African Charismatics: Current Developments within Independent Indigenous Pentecostalism in Ghana* (Leiden: Brill, 2005).

BasicNeeds, *Charting an Economic Revival for People with Mental Illness and Epilepsy,* (Accra, Ghana: BasicNeeds, Ghana/European Commission, 2010).

BasicNeeds, Ghana and Mwananchi, *Ghana: A Picture of Mental Health* (Accra, Ghana: BasicNeeds, Ghana, 2011).

Bediako, Kwame, *Jesus in Africa; The Christian Gospel in African History and Experience* (UK: Regnum Africa, 2000)/(Yaounde, Cameroun: Editions Cle/Akropong-Akuapem, Ghana: Regnum Africa, in association with Paternoster Publishers, UK, 2000).

_____, *Theology and Identity: The Impact of Culture upon Christian Thought in the Second Century and in Modern Africa* (UK: Regnum Books, 1992).

Berinyuu, Abraham A., *Pastoral Care to the Sick in Africa: An Approach to Pastoral Trans-Cultural Theology*, (Frankfurt: Peter Lang, Studies in the Intercultural History of Christianity, Vol. 51; Date of Publication not stated).

Blue, Timothy R., *Compelled: A Memoir of OCD, Anxiety, Depression, Bi-Polar Disorder and Faith...Sometimes* (United States of America, 2012).

Boulaga, Eboussi F, *Christianity Without Fetishes: An African Critique and Recapture of Christianity* (Maryknoll, New York: Orbis Books, 1984).

Bowman, C. and Kuenyehia, A., *Women and Law in Sub-Saharan Africa* (Accra, Ghana: Sedco Publishing, 2003).

Brizendine, Louann, *The Female Brain* (USA: Harmony Books/Crown Publishing Group, 2006).

Bromiley, G.W. (Gen. ed), *The International Standard Bible Encyclopaedia,* Vol. One (Grand Rapids, MI: W.B. Eerdmans Publishing, 1979).

Burt, Vivien K. and Victoria C. Hendrick, *Clinical Manual of Women's Mental Health* (Washington, D.C, USA: American Psychiatric Publishing, Inc., 2005).

Carlson, Dwight L., *Why Do Christians Shoot Their Wounded? Helping (Not Hurting) Those With Emotional Problems* (USA: InterVarsity Press, 1994).

Carmichael, Amy, *You Are My Hiding Place* (Devotional Readings arranged by David Hazard), (USA: Bethany House Publishers, 1991).

Ciarrocchi, Joseph, *A Minister's Handbook of Mental Disorders* (New York: Integration Books, 1993).

Clinebell, Howard J., *The Mental Health Ministry of the Local Church* (Nashville, TN: Abingdon Press, 1965, 1972).

Coker-Appiah, D. and K. Cusack (eds.), *Violence against Women and Children in Ghana* (Ghana, Accra: Gender Studies and Human Rights Documentation Center, 1999).

Collins, Gary, *Christian Counseling: A Comprehensive Guide* (Nashville, TN: Thomas Nelson Publishers, 2007).

Cooper-White, Pamela, *'Many Voices': Pastoral Psychotherapy in Relational and Theological Perspective* (Minnesota: Fortress Press, 2007).

Crabb, Jim and Emma Razi, *Essential Skills for Mental Health Care* (UK: BasicNeeds, Basic Rights, 2007).

Crabb, Larry, *Effective Biblical Counseling: A Model for Helping Caring Christians Become Capable Counselors* (Grand Rapids, Michigan: Zondervan Publishing House, 1977).

Creswell, John W., *Research Design: Qualitative, Quantitative and Mixed Methods Approaches* (Los Angeles, USA: Sage Publications Inc., 2009).

Cusack, Kathy and Takyiwaa Manuh (eds.), *The Architecture of Violence against Women in Ghana* (Ghana, Accra: Gender Studies and Human Rights Documentation Center, 2009).

Dah, Ini Dorcas, *Women Do More Work than Men: Birifor Women as*

Change Agents in the Mission and Expansion of the Church in West Africa (Burkina Faso, Cote d'Ivoire, and Ghana) (Oregon, USA: Wipf and Stock, 2018).

Drogus, Carol Ann, *Women, Religion and Social Change in Brazil's Popular Church* (Indiana: Notre Dame Press, 1979).

Dwamena-Aboagye, Angela, *Thoughts of God: Reflections Before the Desert Storm and Poems from the Wilderness of Hope* (USA: Xulon Press, 2011).

Dwamena-Aboagye, A., Violet E. Awotwi, B. Martin, R. Giordano and K. Polich (eds.), *The CRC-WISE Collaboration Project: Working with Survivors of Gender-Based Violence* (Ghana, Accra: The Ark Foundation and Women's Initiative for Self-Empowerment/M&N Publishing, Accra, 2001).

Eisen, Ute E., *Women Officeholders in Early Christianity: Epigraphical and Literary Studies* (Minnesota: The Liturgical Press, 2000).

Englund, Harry (ed.), *Christianity and Public Culture in Africa* (Ohio: Ohio University Press, 2011).

Entwistle, David N., *Integrative Approaches to Psychology and Christianity: An Introduction to Worldview Issues, Philosophical Foundations and Models of Integration*, 2nd Edition (Eugene, OR: Cascade Books/Wipf and Stock Publishers, 2010).

Eshun, Susan and R.A.R. Gurung (eds.), *Culture and Mental Health: Sociocultural Influences, Theory and Practice* (UK: Blackwell Publishing Ltd, 2009).

Greene-McCreight, Kathryn, *Darkness is My Only Companion: A Christian Response to Mental Illness* (Grand Rapids, Michigan: Brazos Press, 2006).

Hales, Robert E., Stuart. C. Yudofsky and John A. Talbot, *Textbook of Psychiatry*, 2nd Edition (Washington, D.C/London: American Psychiatry Press, 1994).

Hergenhahn, B.R., An *Introduction to the History of Psychology* (USA: Wadsworth Inc., 1986).

Howell, Allison M., *The Religious Itinerary of a Ghanaian People: The Kasena and the Christian Gospel* (Ghana, Accra: African Christian Press, 2001).

Human Rights Watch Report, *'Like a Death Sentence': Abuses against Persons with Mental Disabilities in Ghana* (USA: Human Rights Watch, 2012).

Johnson, Brad W., and William L. Johnson, *The Pastor's Guide to Psychological Disorders and Treatments* (USA: The Hawthorne Press, 2000).

Johnson, Eric L. (ed.), *Psychology and Christianity,* 2nd Edition (Downers Grove, Illinois: InterVarsity Press, 2000).

Karkkainen, Veli-Matti (ed.), *The Spirit in the World: Emerging Pentecostal Theologies in Global Contexts* (Grand Rapids, MI: William B. Eerdmanns Publishing Co., 2009).

Kehoe, Nancy, *Wrestling with our Inner Angels: Faith, Mental Illness and the Journey to Wholeness* (San Francisco, CA: Jossey-Bass, John Wiley and Sons, 2009).

Kendall, R.T., *The Thorn in the Flesh: Hope for All Who Struggle With Impossible Conditions* (Great Britain: Hodder and Stoughton, 1999).

Koenig, Harold G., *Faith and Mental Health: Religious Resources for Healing* (Philadelphia and London: Templeton Foundation Press, 2005).

Kohlenberger III, John R. and James A. Swanson, *The Hebrew English Concordance To The Old Testament, With The New International Version* (Grand Rapids, Michigan: Zondervan Publishing House, c1998).

Kornstein, Susan, G. and Anita H. Clayton (eds.), *Women's Mental Health, A Comprehensive Textbook* (New York: The Guildford Press, 2002).

Kraft, Charles H., *Christianity in Culture: A Study in Dynamic Biblical Theologizing in Cross-Cultural Perspective* (Maryknoll, New York: Orbis Books, 1992).

Krug E.G., L.L. Dahlberg, J.A. Mercy, A.B. Zwi, R. Lozano (eds.), *World Report on Violence and Health* (Geneva: World Health Organization, 2002).

Kuenyehia, Akua (ed.), *Women and Law in West Africa: Situational Analysis of Some Key Issues Affecting Women* (Accra, Ghana: Yamen's Printing and Packaging/WaLWA, Faculty of Law, University of Ghana, 1998).

Kuma, Afua, *Kwaeberentuw ase Yesu* (Ghana: Asempa Publishers, 1981).

Lartey, Emmanuel Y., *In Living Colour: An Intercultural Approach to Pastoral Care and Counselling* (London, UK: Cassell, 1997).

Leach, F., V. Fiscian, E. Kadzamira, E. Lemani, and P. Machakanja, *An Investigative Study of the Abuse of Girls in African Schools* (UK: Department for International Development (DFID), 2003).

Legrand, Lucien, *The Bible on Culture* (Maryknoll, New York, USA: Orbis Books, 2000).

Levin, Bruce L. and Marian A. Becker (eds.), *A Public Health Perspective of Women's Mental Health* (New York: Springer Science+ Business Media LLC Publication, 2010).

Loewenthal, Kate, *Religion, Culture and Mental Health* (Cambridge: Cambridge University Press, 2006).

Luzbetak, Louis L., *The Church and Cultures: New Perspectives in Missiological Anthropology* (Maryknoll, New York: Orbis Books, 2000).

Mandell, Betty R., and Barbara Schram, *Introduction to Human Services, Policy and Practice,* 7th Edition (Boston: Pearson Education Inc., 1997, 2002, 2006, 2009).

Maves, Paul, B. (ed.), *Churches and Mental Health* (New York/London: Charles Scribner and Sons, 1953).

May, Gerald, *Simply Sane: The Spirituality of Mental Health* (New York: The Crossroad Publishing Co., 1977).

Mbiti, John S., *African Religions and Philosophy,* 2nd Edition (London: Heinemann Educational Books Ltd., 1989).

McCann, Richard V., *The Churches and Mental Health* (New York: Basic Books, 1962).

McMinn, Mark R., *Psychology, Theology and Spirituality in Christian Counselling* (Wheaton, Illinois: Tyndale House Publishers, 1996).

McNally, Richard, *What is Mental Illness?* (Cambridge, Massachusetts and London: The Belknap Press of Harvard University Press, 2011).

Mensah, O., J. Williams, R. Atta-Ankomah and M. Mjomba, *Contextual Analysis of the Disability Situation in Ghana* (Accra, Ghana: JMK Consulting, 2008): 31-2, at http://www.gfdgh.org/ Context%20analysis.pdf, accessed 23 May 2016.

Meyer, Birgit, *Translating the Devil: Religion and Modernity among the Ewe in Ghana* (Edinburgh: Edinburgh Press for the International African Institute, 1999).

Milingo, E., *The World in Between: Christian Healing and the Struggle for Spiritual Survival* (London: Hurst and Co., 1984).

Minkah-Premo, S., *Coping with Violence Against Women* (Accra, Ghana: Asempa Publishers, 2001).

Neuger, Christie C., *Counselling Women: A Narrative, Pastoral Approach* (Minnesota: Fortress Press, 2001).

Niebuhr, Richard H., *Christ and Culture* (New York: Harper and Brothers Publishers, 1953).

Nolen-Hoeksema, Susan, *Abnormal Psychology,* 6th Edition (New York, USA: McGraw-Hill Education, 2014).

Oates, Wayne E., *Religious Factors in Mental Illness* (New York: Association Press, 1955).

Oduyoye, Mercy A., *Daughters of Anowa: African Women and Patriarchy* (Maryknoll, New York: Orbis Books, 1995).

Okorocha, Cyril C., *The Meaning of Religious Conversion in Africa: The Case of the Igbo of Nigeria* (USA/UK/Hong Kong: Avebury/Gower Publishing Company Ltd, 1987).

Olupona, Jacob and Sleyman Nyang, *Religious Plurality in Africa:*

Essays in Honour of John S. Mbiti (Berlin: Mouton de Gruyter, 1993).

Onyinah, Opoku, *Pentecostal Exorcism: Witchcraft and Demonology in Ghana* (Dorset, UK: Deo Publishing, 2012).

_____, *Spiritual Warfare: A Centre for Pentecostal Theology Short Introduction* (Cleveland, USA: CPT Press, 2012).

Oppong, C., *Middle Class African Marriage* (UK, London: George Allen and Unwin Publishers, 1981).

Patel, Vikram, *Where There Is No Psychiatrist* (Glasgow, UK: Bell and Bain Ltd/Gaskell, 2013).

Patton, John, *Pastoral Care: The Essential Guide* (Nashville, TN: Abingdon Press, 2005).

Phares, E.J., *Clinical Psychology: Concepts, Methods and Profession*, Revised Edition (USA: The Dorsey Press, 1979, 1984).

Prior, Pauline, *Gender and Mental Health* (New York, USA: New York University Press, 1999).

Renzetti, C.M., J.L. Edleson, R.K. Bergen (eds.), *Sourcebook on Violence Against Women* (California, USA: Sage Publications, 2001).

Republic of Ghana/International Development Institute/Ghana Statistical Service and Associates, *Domestic Violence in Ghana: Incidence, Attitudes, Determinants and Consequences* (UK, Brighton: IDS, 2016).

Romans, Sarah E., and Mary V. Seeman, *Women's Mental Health: A Life-Cycle Approach* (Philadelphia, USA: Lippincott, Williams and Wilkins, 2006).

Rothblum, Esther D. and Ellen Cole (eds.), *Women's Mental Health in Africa* (London: The Haworth Press Inc., 1990).

Shorter, Aylward W.F. (ed.), *African Christian Spirituality* (New York: Orbis Books, Maryknoll, 1978).

Simpson, Amy, *Troubled Minds: Mental Illness and the Church's Mission* (Downers Grove, Illinois: InterVarsity Press, 2013).

Sipe, Richard, A.W. and Clarence J. Rowe (eds.), *Psychiatry, Ministry and Pastoral Counselling* (Collegeville, Minnesota: The Liturgical Press, 1984).

Slater, Lauren, Jessica D. Henderson and Amy E. Banks, *The Complete Guide to Mental Health for Women* (USA, Boston: Beacon Press, 2003).

Smith, Pamela, *Mental Health Care in Settings where Mental Resources are limited: An Easy-Reference Guidebook for Health Care Providers in Developed and Developing Countries* (USA: Archway Publishing, 2014), at www.globalfamilydoctor.com/site/.../MHGuidebook.EBook Download.pdf, accessed 15 February 2014.

Spencer, Aida Besancon and William D. Spencer, *Joy Through the Night: Biblical Resources on Suffering* (Eugene, Oregon: Wipf and Stock

Publishers, 1994).

Stanford, Matthew S., *Grace for the Afflicted: Viewing Mental Illness through the Eyes of Faith* (Colorado Springs, USA: Biblica Publishing, 2008).

Stinton, Diane B. (ed.), *African Theology on the Way: Current Conversations* (London, UK: SPCK Publishing, 2010)

Tanner, Kathryn, *Theories of Culture: A New Agenda for Theology* (Minneapolis: Fortress Press, 1997).

Tew, Jerry (ed.), *Developing Social Models to Understand and Work with Mental Distress* (London and Philadelphia: Jessica Kingsley Publishers, 2002).

The Coalition for the Women's Manifesto for Ghana/Abantu for Development, *The Women's Manifesto for Ghana* (Accra, Ghana: Abantu for Development, 2004).

Toews, John with Eleanor Loewen, *No Longer Alone: Mental Health and the Church* (Waterloo, Ontario: Herald Press, 1995).

Tucker, Ruth and Walter Liefeld, *Daughters of the Church: Women and Ministry from New Testament Times to the Present* (Grand Rapids, Michigan: Zondervan Publishing House, 1987).

VanCleve, Mitzi, *Strivings Within - The OCD Christian: Overcoming Doubt in the Storm of Anxiety* (USA: Goodreads Inc. 2013).

Vine, W.E., *An Expository Dictionary of New Testament Words: With the Precise Meaning for English Readers* (New Jersey, USA: Fleming H. Revell Company, 1966).

Vine, W.E, Merril F. Unger, and William White, *Vine's Complete Expository Dictionary of Old and New Testament Words* (England: Thomas Nelson Publishers, 1984, 1996).

Walls, Andrew F., *The Missionary Movement in Christian History: Studies in the Transmission of Faith* (Edinburgh, Scotland: T &T Clark/ Maryknoll, New York: Orbis Books, 2009).

_____, *The Cross-Cultural Process in Christian History: Studies in the Transmission and Appropriation of Faith* (Maryknoll, New York: Orbis Books, 2002).

Walls, Andrew F. and Cathy Ross (eds.), *Mission in the 21st Century: Exploring the Five Marks of Global Mission* (Maryknoll, New York: Orbis Books, 2008).

Walsh, Sheila, *Loved Back to Life: How I Found the Courage to Live Free* (Nashville, Tennessee: Nelson Books, 2015).

Watts, Fraser, Rebecca Nye and Sarah Savage, *Psychology for Christian Ministry* (London: Routledge Publishers, 2002).

Waruta, D.W. and H.W. Kinoti (eds.), *Pastoral Care in African*

Christianity: Challenging Essays in Pastoral Theology (Action Publishers, Kenya, 1994).

Wield, Cathy, *A Thorn in my Mind: Mental Illness, Stigma and the Church* (Watford, Herts, UK: Instant Apostle, 2012).

Wilkinson, John, *The Bible and Healing: A Medical and Theological Commentary* (Edinburgh: The Handsel Press Ltd, 1998).

World Health Organization, *WHO Multi-Country Study on Women's Health and Domestic Violence Against Women* (Geneva: World Health Organization, 2005).

World Health Organization, *The Mental Health Context: Mental Health Policy and Service Guidance Package* (Geneva: WHO, 2003), at www.who. int/mental_health/policy/services/3_ Context_WEB_07.pdf, accessed 15 February 2016.

Journals, Articles and Manuscripts

Adjetey, Fitnat N.A., 'Religious and Cultural Rights: Reclaiming the African Woman's Individuality – the Struggle between Women's Reproductive Autonomy and African Society and Culture', in Johanna Bond, *Voices of African Women* (USA, North Carolina, Carolina Academic Press, 2004): 274-287.

Ampofo, Adomako A., E. Awotwi, and A. Dwamena-Aboagye, 'How the Perpetrators of Violence Against Women and Children Escape: A Study of "escapes" from the time of the Violent Act, through a Formal Complaint, to Prosecution', in Association of African Women for Research and Development (AAWORD), *Women and Violence in Africa/Femmes et Violences en Afrique* (Ouagadougou, Burkina Faso: Cinquieme Publication, 2005): 216-250.

Amoah, Elizabeth and M.A. Oduyoye, 'The Christ of African Women,' in Virginia Fabella and Mercy Amba Oduyoye, *With Passion and Compassion, Third World Women Doing Theology* (Maryknoll, New York: Orbis Books, 1990 (c 1988): 35-46 (43).

Asamoah-Gyadu, J. Kwabena, 'Drinking from Our Own Wells: The Primal Imagination and Christian Religious Innovation in Contemporary Africa', *Journal of African Christian Thought (JACT)*, Vol. 11, No. 2 (December 2008): 34-42

Awolalu, J.O., 'What is African Traditional Religion?', *Studies in Comparative Religion*, Vol. 10, No. 2 (Spring 1976), at www. studiesincomparativereligion.com, accessed 1 March, 2017.

Bediako, G.M. 'Primal Religion and Christian Faith: Antagonists or Soul Mates?', *Journal of African Christian Thought*, Vol. 3, No. 1 (June 2006): 12-16.

Bediako, Kwame, 'Scripture as the hermeneutic of culture and tradition', *Journal of African Christian Thought*, Vol. 4, No. 1 (June 2001).

Beitman, Benard D., 'Pastoral Counseling Centers: A Challenge to Community Mental Health Centers', *Hospital and Community Psychiatry*, Vol. 33, No. 6 (June 1982): 486-487.

Bergin, Allen, E., 'Values and Religious Issues in Psychotherapy and Mental Health', *American Psychologist*, Vol. 46, No. 4 (April 1991): 394-403, at http://search.proquest.com/docview/ 614392632/ fulltextpdf/1402154C3DOA9F7668/41, accessed 26 August 2013.

Blanch, Andrea, 'Integrating Religion and Spirituality in Mental Health: The Promise and the Challenge', *Psychiatric Rehabilitation Journal*, Vol. 30, No. 4 (2007): 251-260, at http://search. proquest.com/docview/124746327/ fulltextpdf/1402154C3DOA9F7668/5, accessed 26 August 2013.

Blazer, Dan J., 'Religion, Spirituality and Mental Health: What We Know and Why This is a Tough Topic to Research', *Canadian Journal of Psychiatry*, Vol. 54, No. 5 (May 2009): 281-282, at http://search.proquest. com/docview/2222861307/fulltextpdf/1402154C3DOA9F7668/11, 26 August 2013.

Bortei-Doku, E. and A. Kuenyehia, 'Violence Against Women in Ghana', in Kuenyehia. A., (Ed.), *Women and Law in West Africa: Situational Analysis of some Key Issues Affecting Women* (Ghana: Law Faculty, University of Ghana/Yamens Printing and Packaging Ltd., 1998): 272-299.

Bruce, Cuthbert and Thomas, Insel, 'Classification of Issues in Women's Mental Health: Clinical Utility and Etiological Mechanisms', *Archives of Women's Mental Health*, Vol. 13, (2010): 57-59, at http://search.proquest. com/195064233/, 26 August 2013.

Caracci, Giovanni, 'Violence Against Women: Mental Health and the United Nations', *International Journal of Mental Health*, Vol. 32, No. 1, Addressing Global Issues on Violence and Mental Health (Spring 2003): 36-53, at *http://www.jstor.org/stable/41345044, accessed 11 April 2013.*

Carey, Lindsey B. and Laura D. Medico, 'Chaplaincy in Mental Health Care in Aotearoa, New Zealand: An Exploratory Study', *Journal of Religion and Health*, Vol. 52, No. 1 (March 2013), at http://link.springer.com/content/ pdf/10.1007%2Fs/0943-012-9622.pdf, 26 August 2013.

Carrol, H.D.R. and Nana Ama Ofori-Atta, 'Violence against Women in the Gambia', in A. Kuenyehia (ed.), *Women and Law in West Africa: Situational Analysis of some Key Issues Affecting Women* (Ghana: Law Faculty, University of Ghana/Yamens Printing and Packaging Ltd., 1998), pp. 250-271.

Chidarike, Shephard, 'Spirituality: The Neglected Dimension of Holistic Mental Healthcare', *Advances in Mental Health*, Vol. 10, No. 3 (June 2012), pp. 298-302.

Condon, John, 'Women's Mental Health: A "Wish-List" for DSM V', *Archives of Women's Mental Health*, Vol. B1 (February 2010): 5-10, at http://search.proquest.com/docview/19506 3878/fulltextpdf/140288EF3D4C488F/6, accessed 26 August 2013.

de Menil, V., A. Osei, N. Douptcheva, A.G. Hill, P. Yaro and A. De-Graft Aikins, 'Symptoms of Common Mental Disorders and their Correlates among Women in Accra, Ghana: A Population-Based Survey', *Ghana Medical Journal*, Vol. 46, No. 2 (June 2012): 95-103.

'Declaration on Mental Health in Africa: Moving to Implementation', *Global Health Action*, Vol. 7 (2014), pp.4-7, at www.globalhealthaction.net. index/php/ghc.article/view/24589/pdf, accessed 9 February 2016.

Doherty, D. Tedstone and O'Doherty, Y. Kartalova, 'Gender and self-reported mental health problems: predicators of help-seeking from a general practitioner', *British Journal of Health Psychology*, Vol. 15, Part 1 (February 2010): 213-228, at www.ncbi.nlu.nih.gov/pmc/articles/ pmc2845878/pdf/ulmss-29221.pdf, accessed 9 February 2016.

Dwamena-Aboagye, A., 'Polygamy, Equality, and the Gender Debate: A Comparative Study of Ghana and the United States', in Bond, Johanna, *Voices of African Women* (North Carolina, USA: Carolina Academic Press, 2004): 190-204.

Dzokoto, Vivian, A., Adams, Glenn, 'Understanding Genital Shrinking Epidemics in West Africa: Koro, Juju or Mass Psychogenic Illness?', *Culture, Medicine and Psychiatry*, Vol. 29, No. 9 (March 2005): 53-78, at http://search.proquest.com/docview/230000558/accountid=9844. 26 August 2013.

El-Khoury, Y. Mai, Mary A. Dutton, Lisa Goldman, L. Engel and Robin J. Belmaric, 'Ethnic Differences in Battered Women's Formal Help-seeking Strategies: A Focus on Health, Mental Health and Spirituality', *Cultural Diversity and Ethnic Minority Psychology*, Vol. 10, No. 4 (November, 2004): 383-393.

Evans-Anfom, E., 'Traditional Medicine in Ghana: Practice, Problems and Prospects', (1984), *17th Series of the J.B. Danquah Memorial Lectures* (Accra, Ghana: Ghana Academy of Arts and Sciences, 1984).

Foster, G.M., 'Disease Etiology in Non-Western Medical Systems', *Journal of Beliefs and Ethno-Medical Systems*, (1976): 110-117, at http://web.mnstate.edu/robertsb/306/Disease%20 Etiologies %20in%20Non%20 Western%20Medical%20Systems.pdf, accessed 9 March 2017.

Gbedemah, H.A., 'Trokosi: Twentieth Century Female Bondage – A

Ghanaian Case Study', in Bond, Johanna, *Voices of African Women* (North Carolina: USA, Carolina Academic Press, 2004): 83-95.

Grotberg, Edith H., 'Mental Health Aspects of Zar for Women in Sudan', *Women and Therapy*, Vol. 10, No. 3 (3 November 1990): 15, at http://search. proquest.com/216248781?accountid-9844, 26 August 2013.

Guarnaccia, Peter J. and Lloyd H Rogler, 'Research on Culture-Bound Syndromes: New Directions' in *American Journal of Psychiatry*, Vol. 156, 1999: 1322-1327, at http://ajp. psychiatryonline.org/article. aspx?articleid=173679, 29 August 2013.

Gulcur, Leyla, 'Evaluating the Role of Gender Inequalities and Rights Violations in Women's Mental Health', *Health and Human Rights*, Vol. 5, No. 1 (2000), pp. 46-66 at http://www.jstor.org/stable/4065222, accessed 11 April 2013.

Hedelin, Birgitta, and Magaretha Strandmark, 'The Meaning of Mental Health from Elderly Women's Perspectives: A Basis for Health Promotion', *Perspectives in Psychiatric Care* (January-March 2001): 7-14, at http://search. proquest.com/docview/200754937/fulltextpdf /1402112D35174B4FC10/4, accessed 26 August 2013.

Henrica Jansen, A.F.M., L. Heise, C. Watts and C. Garcia-Moreno, 'Intimate Partner Violence and Women's Mental Health, in WHO Multi-Country Study on Women's Health and Domestic Violence: An Observational Study', *The Lancet*, Vol. 371, No. 9619 (April 5-April 11, 2008), pp. 1165-72, at http://searchproquest.com/docview/199019209/ fulltextpdf/140211D35174B4FC10/1, accessed 26 August 2013.

Hodge, David, R., Stephanie E. Moser and S. Michael, 'Spirituality and Mental Health among Homeless Mothers', *Social Work Research*, Vol. 36, No. 4 (December, 2012): 245-255, at http://search.proquest.com/1288749727/.

Howell, Allison, 'Prisca, Maxmilla and Madam Karuwu: Insights into Women Prophets of the Second Century Church and Twentieth Century African Christianity', *JACT*, Vol. 13, No. 1 (June 2010): 35-44.

Idowu, Bolaji 'The Predicament of the Church in Africa', in C.G. Baëta (ed.), *Christianity in Tropical Africa*.

Jansen, Henrica, A.F.M., Lori Heise, Charlotte H. Watts and Claudia, Garcia-Moreno, 'Intimate Partner Violence and Women's Mental Health in the WHO Multi-Country Study on Women's Health and Domestic Violence: An Observational Study', *The Lancet*, Vol. 371, No. 9619 (5-11 April 2008): 1165-72, at http://search.proquest.com/docview/199019209/fulltextpdf/ 1402112D35174B4FC10/1, accessed 26 August 2013.

Kastrup, Marianne, 'War and women mental health', *World Cultural Psychiatry Research* Review, Vol. 1, No. 4 (2006): 29-33, at https://www.

wcprr.org/wp-content/uploads/2013/09/ jan0629332.pdf, accessed 25 February 2017.

Khumalo, I.P., Q.M. Temane and M.P Wissing, 'Socio-Demographic Variables, General Psychological Well-Being and the Mental Health Continuum in an African Context.' *Social Indicators Research*, Vol. 105, No. 3 (February, 2012): 419-442, at http://search/proquest.com/ docview/913337049/ fulltextpdf/14021BAD180A10FDAD/1, 26 August 2013.

King, Dana, E., D. Cubmings and L. Whelstone, 'Attendance at Religious Services and Subsequent Mental Health in Midlife Women', *International Journal of Psychiatry in Medicine* (2005): 287-297 at http://search.proquest. com/docview/196305121/fulltextpdf/1402112D35174 B4FC10/7, 26 August 2013.

Koenig, Harold, G., 'Religion, Spirituality and Health: The Research and Clinical Implications', *International Scholarly Research Network*, (2012): 1-33, at http://search.proquest.com/docview/ 1272300888/ fulltextpdf/1402154C3D0A9F7668/3, 26 August 2013.

Konopasek, Zdenek, and Jan Palecek, 'Apparitions and Possessions as Boundary Objects: An Exploration into some Tensions between Mental Health Care and Pastoral Care', *Journal on Religion and Health*, Vol. 51, No. 3 (September 2012): 970-985 at http://linkspringer.com/ content/ pdf/10.1007%Fs10943-40-9409-9.pdf, 26 August 2013.

Kosits, Russel, D., 'Whose Psychology? Which Christianity?', *McMaster Journal of Theology and Ministry (MJTM)*, Vol. 12 (2011-2012): 101-195.

Koss, Mary, P., 'The Women's Mental Health Research Agenda: Violence Against Women', *American Psychologist*, Vol. 45, No. 3 (March 1990): 374-380.

Kovess-Masfety, Viviane, Ann Dezelter, Ron de Graaf, Joseph M. Haro, Ronny Bruffaerts et al., *Social Psychiatry and Psychiatric Epidemiology*, Vol. 45, No. 10 (October 2010): 989-998, at http://search.proquest.com/ docview/751419013/fulltextpdf/1402154C3D0A9F7668/75, 26 August 2013.

Kunst, Jennifer, L., 'Christians' Attitudes towards Mental Health Intervention in the Church: An Exploratory Study', *Review of Religious Research*, Vol. 34, No. 3 (March 1993): 225-234 at http://www.jstor.org/ stable/3700596, accessed 11 April 3013.

Larbi, Emmanuel, K., 'The Nature of Continuity and Discontinuity of Ghanaian Pentecostal Concept of Salvation in African Cosmology', *Cyberjournal for Pentecostal Charismatic Research*, at http://www.pctii. org/cyberj/cyberj10/larbi.html, accessed on 30 August 2011.

Larson, Mary Jo, and Sarah McGraw, 'Physical Illness and Medical Needs of Women with Mental Disorders', in Bruce Lobotsky Levin and Marion Ann

Becker (eds.), *A Public Health Perspective of Women's Mental Health*, (New York: SpringerScience +Business Media, LLC, 2010): 81-105.

Laye, Camara. 'The Soul of Africa', in Aylward W.F. Shorter (ed.), *African Spirituality* (New York: Orbis Books, Maryknoll, 1978).

Levin, Jeff, 'Religion and mental health: Theory and Research', *International Journal of Applied Psychoanalytic Studies Online* (2010), at www.interscience.wiley.com/D01:10.1002/aps.240, accessed 15 February 2016.

Maclean, Faith, 'Mental Health and Justice: The Case of Andreas Yates', *The Lancet,* Vol. 368, Issue 9551, 2 December 2006: 1951-1954, at www.thelancet.com/journals/lancet/ articles/PIISO140-6736(06)69789-4/fulltext, 9 September 2013.

Magoke-Mhoja, M.E., 'Impact of Customary Inheritance on the Status of Widows and Daughters in Tanzania: A Challenge to Human Rights Activists', in Johanna Bond, *Voices of African Women* (USA, North Carolina, Carolina Academic Press, 2004): 255-266.

Manasseh, Elizabeth Leelavathi, 'Women and Violence', in Beulah Wood (ed.), *Side by Side: Gender from a Christian Perspective* (Bangalore, India: SAIACS Press, 2007): 189-203.

Manuh, Takyiwaa and A. Dwamena-Aboagye, 'Implementing Domestic Violence Legislation in Ghana: The Role of Institutions', in Mulki Al Sharmani (ed.), *Feminist Activism, Women's Rights, and Legal Reform* (London, UK: Zed Books Ltd, 2013): 203-234.

Maracek, Jeanne and Deborah J. Ballou, 'Family Roles and Women's Mental Health,' Professional Psychology, Vol. 12, No. 1 (February 1981): 39-46, at http://search.proquest.com/ docview/1614290811/..., accessed 26 August 2013.

Mastekaasa, Arne, 'Marital Status, Distress and Well-Being: An International Comparison', *Journal of Comparative Family Studies*, Vol. 24, No. 2 (Summer 1994): 185-205 at http://www.jstor.org/stable/41602320 , accessed 11 April 2013.

McBride, Angela, B., 'Mental Health Effects of Women's Multiple Roles', *America Psychologist*, Vol. 45, No. 3 (March 1009): 381-384, at http://search.proquest.com/docview/ 614273162/fulltextpdf/1402112D35174B4FC10/1, accessed 26 August 2013.

Mengesha, Maigerete and Earlise C. Ward, 'Psychotherapy with African-American women with depression: Is it okay to talk about their religious/spiritual beliefs?', *Religions*, Vol. 3, (2012), pp. 19-36, at www.mdpi.com/journal/religions, accessed 26th August, 2013.

Meyer, Birgit, 'Going and Making Public: Pentecostalism as Public

Religion in Ghana', in Englund, Harry, (Ed), *Christianity and Public Culture in Africa* (Ohio: Ohio University Press, 2011), pp. 149-166.

Morris, Cerise, 'Mental Health Matters: Towards a Non-Medicalised Approach to Psychotherapy with Women', *Women and Therapy*, Vol. 20, No. 3 (1997): 63-77, at http://search.proquest.com/ docview/216249352/ fulltextpdf/1402112D35174B4FC10/1, 26 August 2013.

Morrison, Ian, 'Pastoral Care and Mental Health: An Anglican Minister's Perspective', Australian *Journal of Pastoral Care and Health*, Vol. 2, No. 2 (December 2008), at http://www.pastoral journal.findus.com/pdfs/Health. pdf, 17 July 2013.

Mwuara, P.N., 'Unsung Bearers of Good News: AIC Women and the Transformation of Society in Africa', *Journal of African Christian Theology*, Vol. 7, No. 1 (June 2004): 38-44.

Nwoye, Augustine, 'Hope-Healing Communities in Contemporary Africa', *The Journal of Humanistic Psychology*, Vol. 42, No. 4 (Fall 2002): 58-81, at http://jhp.sagepub.com/content /42/4/58, 26 August 2013.

Ofori-Atta, A., S. Cooper, B. Akpalu, A. Osei, V. Doku, C. Lund, A. Fisher and the MHAPP Research Project Consortium 'Common Understandings of women's mental illness in Ghana: Results from a qualitative study', *International Review of Psychiatry*, Vol. 6, No. 22 (2010): 589-598, at http:// r4d.dfid.gov.uk/pdf/outputs/mentalhealth_rpc/ofori-attaetal_intrevpsy2010. pdf, accessed 17 June 2016.

Ofori-Boadu, Gloria. 'Ghanaian Women, Law and Economic Power', in Johanna Bond, *Voices of African Women* (USA, North Carolina, Carolina Academic Press, 2004): 349-365.

Osei, O. Akwasi, 'Witchcraft and depression: A study into the psychopathological features of alleged witches', *Ghana Medical Journal*, Vol. 35, No. 3: 111-115.

Parsitau, Damaris, '"Arise Oh Ye Daughters of Faith": Women, Pentecostalism and Public Culture in Kenya', in Harry Englund (ed.), *Christianity and Public Culture in Africa* (Ohio: Ohia University Press, 2011): 131-145.

Patel, Vibhuti, 'Women's Right to Mental Health', *Journal of Psychosocial Research*, Vol. 5, No. 2 (2010): 275-281, at http://search. proquest.com/docviw/1862714149/fulltextpdf/142112D35174 B4FC10/1, accessed 26 August 2013.

Patel, Vikram and Arthur Kleinman, 'Poverty and common mental disorders in developing countries', *Bulletin of the World Health Organization (WHO)*, Vol. 81, No. 8, (2003): 609-615, at www.who.int/bulletin/ volumes/81/8/Patel0803.pdf, accessed 9 February 2016.

Patel, Vikram, 'Mental health in low and middle income countries', *British Medical Bulletin,* Vol. 81, No. 81 (2007): 81-96, at www.http://bmb. oxfordjournals.org/content/81-82/81full.pdf, accessed 9 February 2016.

Patel, Vikram and Norman Sartorius, 'From science to action: The Lancet Series on Global Mental Health', *Current Opinion in Psychiatry,* Vol. 21 (2008), at www.http://psychiatry.utoronto.ca/wp-Content/uploads/2012/13/ Patel-Sartorius-2008-overview-of-lancet-2007-series.pdf, accessed 9 February 2016.

Pathare, Saumitra and Laura S. Shields, 'Supported Decision-Making for Persons with Mental Illness: A Review', *Public Health Reviews,* Vol. 34, No. 2 (2012): 1-40 (3-4), at www.publichealthreviews.eu/uploads/pdf_files/12/00_ pathare.pdf, accessed 25 August 2012.

Price, Michael, 'Study finds some significant differences in brains of men and women', *Referred Academic Journal,* 11 April 2017, at http://www. sciencemag.org/news/2017/04/study-finds-significant-differences-brains-men-and-women, accessed 22 July 2017.

Read, U.M. and V.C.K. Doku, 'Mental health research in Ghana: A Literature Review', *Ghana Medical Journal,* Vol. 46, No. 2 (June 2012) at www.ncbi.nim.nih.gov/pmc/articles/PMC_3645145/pdf/GM/4625-0029.pdf, accessed 17 June 2016.

Ross, Alistair, 'The future of Pastoral Counselling', *Whitefield Briefing,* Vol. 1, No. 2 (9 March 1996): 1-4, at www.klice.co.uk/uploads/whitfield/ vol%201.2%20Ross%20.pdf, accessed 3 March 2016.

Sam, Bernice, 'Discrimination in the Traditional Marriage and Divorce System in Ghana: Looking at the Problem from a Human Rights Perspective', in Bond, Johanna, *Voices of African Women: Women's Rights in Ghana, Uganda and Tanzania* (North Carolina, USA: Carolina Academic Press, 2005): 205-217.

Schneider, Renne, Nikki Baumrind and Rachel Kimmering, 'Exposure to Child Abuse and Risk for Mental Health Problems in Women', *Violence and Victims,* Vol. 22, No. 5 (2007): 620-631, at http://search.proquest. com/docview/208556802/fulltextpdf/140288E2AF3D4C488F/5, accessed 26 August 2013.

Sefa-Dedeh, A., 'Religion and Psychotherapy', in Angela Ofori-Atta and Samuel Ohene (eds.), *Changing Trends in Mental Health Care and Research in Ghana: A Reader of the Department of Psychiatry, University of Ghana Medical School* (Accra, Ghana: University Press, 2014).

Shepard, L.D., 'The Impact of Polygamy on Women's Mental Health: A Systematic Review', *Epidemiology and Psychiatric Sciences,* Vol. 22, Issue 01 (March 2013): 47-62, at http:// journals.cambridge.org/download.php/

file=%2f10968-F1789FOF9486DA1502071B, 26 August 2013.

Sipsma, Heather, Angela Ofori-Atta, Maureen Canavan, Isaac Osei-Akoto, Christopher Udry and Elizabeth H., Bradley, 'Poor mental health in Ghana: Who is at risk?' *Bio Med Central* (The Open Access Publisher), 1 April 2013, at www.bmcpublichealth.biomedcentral.com/article/ 10.1186/1471-2458-13-288, accessed 17 June 2016.

Stanford Matthew S. and Kandace R McAlister, 'Perceptions of Serious Mental Illness in a Local Congregation', *Journal of Religion, Disability and Health*, Vol. 12, No. 2, 2008: 144-153, at http://jrdh.haworthpress.com, doi.10.1080/152289060802/60654, accessed, 4 February 2015.

Stansbury, Kim, L., Harley, Debra, A., Kind, Lois, Nelson, Nancy, Speight, Gillian, 'African-American clergy: What are their perceptions of pastoral care and pastoral counseling?', *Journal of Religion and Health*, Vol. 51, Issue 3 (September 2012): 961-969.

Steglitz, Jeremy, Reuben Ng, John Mosho and Trace Kershaw, 'Divinity and Distress: The Impact of Religion and Spirituality on the Mental Health of HIV-Positive Adults in Tanzania', *AIDS and Behavior*, Vol. 16, No. 8 (November 2012): 2392-2398, at http://search.proquest.com/..., accessed 26 August 2013.

Stewart, D.E., M. Rondon, G. Damiani and J. Honikman, 'International Psycho-Social and Systemic Issues in Women's Mental Health', *Archives of Women's Mental Health*, Vol. 4, No. 1 (November, 2001): 13-17, at http://search.proquest.com/195062437/accountid=9844, accessed 26 August 2013.

Taylor Roberts, J., Christopher G. Ellison, Linda M., Levin Chatters, S. Jeffrey and Karen D. Lincoln, 'Mental Health Services in Faith Communities: The Role of Clergy in Black Churches', *Social Work*, Vol. 45, No. 1 (January 2000): 73-87.

Tertullien: *De Praescriptione Haeriticorum*, 7, 9-13, in Volumes I and II of *Corpus Christianorum, Series Latina* (CCL), Turnhout, 1954.

UNICEF/ Innocenti Research Centre, 'Domestic Violence Against Women and Girls', *Innocenti Digest*, No. 6, May, 2000).

Walls, Andrew F., 'Christian Scholarship in Africa in the Twenty-first Century', *Journal of African Christian Thought*, Vol. 4, No. 2 (December 2001).

Walter, Tony, 'Why are Most Churchgoers Women? A Literature Review', *Vox Evangelica*, Vol. 20 (1990): 73-90 (79) at www.biblicalstudies.org.uk/pdf/vox/vol20/women_walter.pdf, accessed 9 February 2016.

Young, John, Ezra Griffith and David, R. Williams, 'The Integral Role of Pastoral Counseling by African-American Clergy in Community Mental Health', *Psychiatry Services*, Vol. 54, No. 5 (May 2003): 688-692, at http://

ps.psychiatryonline.org/data/journals/pss/4355/688.pdf, accessed 26 August 2013.

Theses, Dissertations and other Research Project Documents

ACTIONAID, 'Condemned without Trial: Women and Witchcraft in Ghana', (September, 2012) at https://ww.actionaid.org.uk/sites/default/files/doc-lib/ghana-report-single-pages.pdf, accessed 6 July 2016.

Cherry, Kendra, 'Psychology Theories', http://psychology.about.com/od/psychology101/u/psy chology-the, 16 August 2013.

Cohen, Andrew, '10 Years Later: The Tragedy of Andreas Yates', *The Atlantic* (11 March 2012), at www.theatlantic.com/national/archives/2012/03, 9 September 2013.

'Cultural Factors in Psychiatric Disorders', at www.mentalhealth.com/magi/wolfgang.html, 23 March 2013.

Dah, Ini Dorcas, 'Birifor Women Communicating the Gospel: An Analysis of the Work and Contributions of Birifor Women to the Growth of the Church in West Africa (Burkina Faso, Cote D'Ivoire and Ghana)', A thesis submitted in partial fulfilment of the requirements for the degree of Doctor of Philosophy, Akrofi-Christaller Institute for Theology, Mission and Culture, Akropong-Akuapem, Ghana, September 2015.

Del-Vecchio, Mary-Jo, 'Women's Mental Health', at http://.un.org/womenwatch/daw/csw/ mental.htm, accessed 17 July 2013.

Denno, Deborah W., 'Who is Andreas Yates? A Short Story About Insanity', at http:// scholarship.law.duke.edu/cgi/viewcontent.cgi, 9 September 2013.

Dwamena-Aboagye, Angela, 'An Analysis of the Hierarchicalist and Egalitarian Debate on Gender Relations in the Western Evangelical Church from the Perspective of an African Christian Woman', A dissertation submitted in fulfilment of a Master-of-Theology degree at Akrofi-Christaller Institute for Theology, Mission and Culture, Akropong-Akuapem, Ghana, 2013.

Evangelical Lutheran Church in America, 'The Body of Christ and Mental Illness: A Social Message adopted by the Church Council', 3 November 2011, at www.elca.org /.../mental_illness.pdf, accessed 15 February 2016.

Feldman, Jackie, M., 'History of Community Psychiatry', Handbook of Community Psychiatry, at http://www.springer.com/978/-/-4614-3/48-0, accessed 15 February 2016.

'Feminist Research', at http://www.palgrave.com/sociology/sarantakos/chapter3.pdf, 15 August 2013.

'Gender Research Methodologies' at http://www.wunrn.com/

news/2008/03_08/03_17_08 /031708_gender.htm, 16 August 2013.

Ghana Statistical Service (GSS), *Socio-Economic and Demographic Trends Analysis, Vol. 1*, (Accra, Ghana: Ghana Statistical Service, 2005), at http://Downloads/ 2000_phc_data_analysis_report_volume_1.pdf, accessed 21 April 2016.

Ghana Statistical Service, *Ghana Living Standards Survey (GLSS Round 6), Main Report* (Government of Ghana (GOG)/DfID/ UNDP/UNICEF/ GSS, 2014), at http://www.gh.undp.org /content/dam/ghana/docs/Doc/ Inclgro/UNDP_GH_IG_2010MDGreport_18102013.pdf, accessed 7 April 2016.

Ghana Statistical Service (GSS), *Women and Men in Ghana - 2010 Population and Housing Census Report* (Accra, Ghana: Ghana Statistical Service, 2013).

Ghana Statistical Service (GSS), *2010 Population and Housing Census - Summary of Final Results* (Accra, Ghana: Sakoa Press Ltd), at http://www. statsghana.gov.gh/docfiles /2010phc/Census2010_Summary_report_of_final_ results.pdf, accessed 23 May 2016.

Government of Ghana and Ministry of Gender, Children and Social Protection (GOG/MoGSCP), *Ghana's Combined Sixth and Seventh Periodic Reports on the Implementation of the United Nations Convention on the Elimination of all forms of Discrimination Against Women (CEDAW)*, (Ghana: Republic of Ghana/MoGSCP, 2011-2015).

Government of Ghana/Ministry of Gender, Children and Social Protection (GOG/MoGSCP, 'Gender Statistics in the Republic of Ghana', A Report presented to the CEDAW Conference, Geneva, by the Minister of Gender Children and Social Protection, Honourable Nana Oye Lithur, (Ghana: GOG/MoGSCP, October, 2014).

Government of Ghana/Ministry of Gender, Children and Social Protection, *National Gender Policy* (Accra, Ghana: Ministry of Gender, Children and Social Protection, 2015).

Glasgow SPCMH, 'Mental Health in Different Cultures', at http:// glasgowsteps.com /facts/cultures.php, 23 March 2013.

Goldstein, Jackie, 'Geel, Belgium: A model of "Community Recovery"', (Samford University Psychology Department, 2009), at http://faculty.Samford. edu~jlgoldst, accessed 10 March 2016.

Green, Judith and Nicki Thorogood, *Qualitative Methods for Health Research* (London/Thousand Oaks/ New Delhi: Sage Publications, 2004), at www.sxf.uevora.pt/wp-content/uploads/ 2013/or/Green_2004.pdf, accessed 3 December 2016.

Hills, D., E. Aram, D. Hinds, C. Warrington, L. Brisett and L. Stock, 'Traditional Healers Action Research Project', Final Report prepared by the

Tavistock Institute of Human Relations (for The King's Fund), London, UK, 13 May 2013.

Horton, Michael S., 'Faith and Mental Illness' at http://www.modernreformation.org/default.php?page=articledisplay&var1=ArtRead&var2=1542&var3=main, accessed 5 April 2014.

Hunter, Gordon M, 'Qualitative Research', at www.people.uleth.ca/~Hunter2.doc, 16 August 2013.

Hurst, Sarah-Louise, 'Church leaders' experience of supporting congregants with mental health difficulties', A Dissertation submitted in partial fulfilment for the degree of Doctor of Clinical Psychology, University of Wales, Cardiff and South Wales Doctoral Course in Clinical Psychology, May 2011.

Icelandic Human Rights Centre, General Comments and UN Facts Sheets: UN Fact Sheet No. 23 – 'Harmful Traditional Practices Affecting the Health of Women and Children', at http://www.humanights.is/the-human-rights-project.../no.23harmful-traditional-practices/, accessed on 6 September 2014.

International Association for Women's Mental Health, www.iawmh.org, 20 August 2013.

Interpersonal Violence Against Women', *World Psychiatry*, Vol. 5, No. 1 (February 2006): 61-4, at http://www.ncbi.nlm.nih.gov/pmc/articles/pmc1472251, 20 August 2013.

'Key Informant Interview', article at http://healthpolicy.ucla.edu/programs/health-data/ trainings/Docu 25 August 2013.

Knobloch, Neil, A. 'Building Conceptual and Theoretical Frameworks that inform Research', at http://www.public.iastate.edu/~loanam/ACTER/2010/symposia/Bril, 16th, August, 2013

Koroma, Karim Kelvin, 'Christian Mission and African Traditional Medicine: Case Studies of Gospel and Culture Engagement', Unpublished dissertation in fulfilment of a Master of Theology (MTh) degree at Akrofi-Christaller Institute of Theology, Mission and Culture, Akropong, Ghana, 2013.

Leduc, Birgitte, 'Guidelines for Gender Sensitive Research', at www.icimod.org/resource/1290, 16 August 2013.

Lester, Stan, 'An Introduction to Phenomenological Research', at http://www.sld.demon .co.uk/resmethy.pdf, 31 July 2013.

LifeWay Research, *Study of Acute Mental Illness and the Christian Faith Research Report* (Undated) at www.lifewayresearch.com/.../Acute-Mental-Illness-and-Christian-Faith-Research, accessed 15 February 2016.

Lives and Legacies, 'Reflexivity: A Process of Reflection', http://www.

utsc.utoronto.ca /~pchsiung/LA/reflexivity, 31 July 2013.

Madeiros, Marcelo, and Joana Costa, 'What do we mean by Feminization of Poverty?', International Poverty Centre, No. 58, July 2008, at www.ipc-undp.org, accessed 1 March 2016.

Melvarez, Silvina, 'Global Perspectives on Mental Health', (2008), at www.ispn.psych.org/docs /GlobalPerspectMentalHealth 0804.pdf, accessed 15 February 2016.

Minson, Robert, H, and Celia P. Minson, 'Models of Christian Counseling, Coaching and Pastoral Care', (2014), A Presentation at Bukai Life Centre, at www.slideshare.net/celiaMinson/models-of-pastora-care-and-counseling, accessed 3 March 2016.

Moultire, Alison and Sharon Kleintjes, 'Women's Mental Health in South Africa', at http://www. hst.org.za/uploads/files/chap21_06.pdf, 15 August 2013.

Nalini, Pandalangat, 'Cultural Influences on Help-Seeking, Treatment and Support for Mental Health Problems: A Comparative Study using a Gender Perspective, A thesis submitted in fulfilment of the degree of Doctor of Philosophy, Institute of Medical Science, University of Toronto, 2011, at http://tspace.library.utoronto.ca/bitstream/1807/31890/3/Pandalongat_Nalini _2011_PhD_thesis, accessed 17 July 2013.

National Development Planning Commission /Government of Ghana (NDPC/GOG), *2010 Report on the Millennium Development Goals*, (Ghana: NDPC/GOG, 2012), at http://www.gh.undp.org/ content/dam/ghana/docs/ Doc/Inclgro/UNDP_GH_IG_2010MDGreport_18102013.pdf, accessed 7 April 2016.

Nwokoro, Samuel, O.N.G., 'The Influence of Traditional Religion on African Christianity', A Lecture presented at Nifes Conference Centre, Abuja, Nigeria on 17 August 2014.

Onyinah, Opoku, 'Akan Witchcraft and the Concept of Exorcism in the Church of Pentecost', A thesis submitted in fulfilment of the requirements for the degree of Doctor of Philosophy, University of Birmingham (February 2002), at www.http://etheses.bham.ac/uk/1694/1/Onyinah 02.PhD.pdf, accessed 11 December 2014.

Osarenren, L., 'Tradition at the Heart of Violence Against Women and Girls in Africa', Pambazuka News, Issue 351, June 3, 2008, at http://www. pambazukanet/en/category/comment /46520, accessed 6 September 2014.

Osei, Joseph, 'The Spirit-Child Phenomenon', at http://www.ghanaweb. com/GhanaHomePage/NewsArchive/The-spirit-child-phenomenon-286693 , (25th Sept, 2013), accessed 17 June 2016.

Patel, Vikram, 'Gender in Mental Health Research', World Health

Organization (WHO) Gender in Mental Health Research Series, (2005), at www. who.int/gender/documents/Mental Healthlast2.pdf, accessed 9 February 2016.

Patton, Michael Q. and Michael Cochran, 'A Guide to using Qualitative Research Methodologies', (2002) at http://evaluation.msf.at/filesadmin/ evaluation/files/documents/ resources-MSF/MSF-Qualitative-Methods.pdf, 31 July 2013.

Platt-McDonald, Sharon, *A Mental Wellness Handbook*, (UK: British Union Conference Health Ministries Department, 2009), at www.http:// adventist.org.uk/...pdf.../Complete-Mental-Wellness-Handbook.pdf, accessed 15 February 2016.

Psychology Dictionary (online), http://psychologydictionary.org, 20 August 2013

Razee, Husna '"Being a Good Woman": Suffering and Distress through the Voice of Women in the Maldives', A thesis submitted in fulfilment of the requirements for the degree of Doctor in Philosophy, School of Public Health and Community Medicine, University of South Wales, Sydney, Australia, (August, 2006), at http://www.unswork.unsw.edu.au/primo_library /lib-web/, 1 August 2013.

Republic of Ghana/Ministry of Gender, Children and Social Protection (MOGSCP), *Ghana National Social Protection Policy* (Accra, Ghana: MOGSCP, December 2015).

Selvam, Sahaya G. 'Positive Psychology as a Theoretical Framework for Studying and Learning about Religion from the Perspective of Psychology', at http://www.academia.edu/1161421/ Positive Psychology_as_a_theoretical_ framework, 16 August 2013.

Spurgeon, Charles, 'The Sick Man Left Behind', Original Sermon from the Sick Room of C.H Spurgeon, Metropolitan Tabernacle Pulpit, No. 1452A, 12 January 1879, at http://www. spurgeongems.org/.../chs1452A. pdf, accessed 1 April 2015.

Sustainable Development Goals, adopted by the UN on 25 September 2015, at www.un.org/sustainable-development/sustainable-development-goals/, accessed 17 June 2016.

Swatos, William, A. (ed), 'Psychology of Religion', *Encyclopedia of Religion and Society*, (California: AltaMira Press, 1998), at http://hirr.hartsem. edu/ency/Psychology.htm, 20 August 2013.

The Culture of Mental Health, in *Psychology Today*, at http:// psychologytoday.com/blog/culture-in mind/2011, 23 March 2013.

The Grace Alliance, http://www.mentalhealthgracealliance.org/mental-illness/eq, 17 July 2013.

'The Historical Approach to Research', from http://www.gslis.utexas. edu/~palmquis/courses/ historical/htm, at http://rmc.ncr.vt.edu/wp-content/

uploads/2008/05/q7-historicalmethodsinfo resources.pdf, 9 September 2013.

The UN Intellectual History Project, 'The UN and Human Development: The Concept of Human Development', at http://hdr.undp.org/en/media/ jolly%/20HDR%/20NOTE5/20%/UN, 16 August 2013.

The Willowbank Report, Report of a Consultation on Gospel and Culture held at Willowbank, Somerset Bridge, Bermuda, 8 -13 January 1978.

The World Bank, 'Maternal Mortality Ratio (modelled estimate, per 100,000 live births, 1990-2015), at www.data.worldbank.org, accessed 17 November 2016.

Twumasi, Patrick, A., 'The Interrelationship between Scientific and Traditional Medical Systems: A Study of Ghana', A thesis submitted to the Department of Sociology, Faculty of Graduate Studies, in partial fulfilment of the requirement for the degree of Doctor of Philosophy, University of Alberta, Edmonton, Canada, 1972.

UNESCO, *The 2009 UNESCO Framework for Cultural Statistics*, (UNESCO, General Conference, 35th Session, 18 September 2009), at www. culturalpolicies.net/web/files/134/ en/FCS_2009.doc, accessed 10 September 2016.

Vaismoradi, M., H. Turunen and T. Bondas, 'Content analysis and thematic analysis: Implications for conducting a qualitative descriptive study', *Nursing and Health Science*, Vol. 15 (2013): 398-405, at www.53e317510cf2b9dod832cb47.pdf, accessed 3 December 2016.

Vassol, Elverta L., 'African American Pastors' Perceptions of their Congregants Mental Health Needs, A dissertation submitted in partial fulfilment of the requirements for the degree of Doctor of Philosophy, Kansa State University, 2005.

Webb, Marcia, 'Towards a Theology of Mental Health', Lecture, 2009 Winifred E. Weter Faculty Award Lecture, Seattle Pacific University, 16 April 2009, at http://www.spu.edu/depts/ csfd/documents/weter, accessed 23 March 2013.

Webb, Marcia, Kathy Stetz and Kristin Heddon, 'Representation of Mental Illness in Christian Self-Help Best Sellers', A Study at Seattle Pacific University, at http://spu.edu/depts/.../ Christianbestsellersstigma/ SPUWebsiteversion.pdf, accessed 15 February 2016.

WHO, 1997 Report, 'Violence against Women: Definition and Scope of the Problem', at www.who.int/gender/violence/v4.pdf, accessed 30 August 2016.

WHO, *The World Health Report, 2001: Mental Health – New Understanding, New Hope* (Geneva: World Health Organization, 2001): 1-17 at www.who.int/whr/2001/en, accessed 22 August 2016.

WHO, (2004b), *Promoting Mental Health – concepts - emerging evidence- practice-summary report* (Geneva: World Health Organization, 2004): 15 at www.who.int/mental_health/evidence /en/promoting_mhh.pdf, accessed 22 August 2016.

Wood, Peter, and Nich Pratt, 'Qualitative Research', at http://www.edu. plymouth.ac.uk/resined/ qualitative%20method, 31 July 2013.

World Health Organization and Ministry of Health, Ghana, *WHO-AIMS Report on Mental Health System in Ghana* (WHO, Accra Office/Africa Region, 2011).

World Psychiatry Association, 'The International Consensus Statement on Women's Mental Health and the World Psychiatry Association Consensus Statement on UN Women', 'The Feminization of Poverty', Fact Sheet No. 1, (United Nations Department of Public Information, May, 2000), at www. un.org, accessed 1 March 2016.